Controlling
PMS

David Hazard

HARVEST HOUSE PUBLISHERS
Eugene, Oregon 97402

Cover by Left Coast Design, Portland, Oregon

Advisory

*Readers are advised to consult with their physician or other
medical practitioner before implementing
the suggestions that follow.
This book is not intended to take the place of sound
medical advice or to treat specific maladies. Neither the author nor
the publisher assumes any liability for possible adverse
consequences as a result of the information contained herein.*

CONTROLLING PMS
Copyright © 2002 by David Hazard
Published by Harvest House Publishers
Eugene, Oregon 97402

ISBN 0-7369-0484-0

Printed in the United States of America.

Contents

Healthy Body, Healthy Soul 5

1. When Life Is a Vicious Cycle 7

2. Cleansing Your Mind. 16

3. Empowering Your Spirit. 30

4. The PMS Diet 47

5. Nature's Apothecary 63

6. Getting Your Body on Your Side 81

7. Finding Balance. 100

Notes. 109

Healthy Body, Healthy Soul

Medical science is now re-discovering something people of faith and wisdom have known for ages: Our physical body and our inner being are amazingly interconnected. In fact, we humans are marvelously designed creations. So taught the psalmist many centuries ago when he described us as "fearfully and wonderfully made."

So close is this connection between our body and our inner being that if *one* part of us is weak or sick, eventually our *whole being* can be affected.

Conversely, whenever we create good health in one aspect of our being it will have positive benefits for our whole person. It only makes sense, then, to address the health problems that plague us—such as PMS—by taking a "whole-person" approach to restoring well-being.

Controlling PMS takes this whole-person approach and offers proven natural healthcare remedies to help control or relieve even the worst symptoms of premenstrual syndrome. The strategies offered are simple and natural…and many have been used for centuries by women dealing with the same distresses you now suffer.

Like the other books in this series, this book is not offered as a substitute for the support you may need from caring professionals, such as a general doctor, gynecologist, psychiatrist, psychological counselor, or member of the clergy.

Nonetheless, ultimately we are each responsible for our own healthcare. And there are many things women can do to overcome or control the symptoms of PMS. For that reason, this book offers a wide range of simple strategies that can supplement your work with a caring professional. In the end, your health *will* benefit.

With this in mind, *Controlling PMS* can help you learn

- mental and spiritual strategies that will de-stress and strengthen you from within

- information about foods that trigger or magnify PMS symptoms…and foods that can actually help minimize them

- up-to-date information about natural supplements— from vitamins and minerals, to herbs and homeopathic remedies—that are helping women cope and heal

- simple and easy ways to get your body back on your side...through rejuvenating workouts and techniques that will physically relax you and relieve distress

This book doesn't offer a "program"—rather, it offers a wide range of options you can try. Some may work for you and fit in with your lifestyle better than others.

Throughout, you will also encounter helpful, informational "sidebars" that will offer even more great, natural ideas to help ease your symptoms and restore well-being. As you find the strategies and remedies that work for you, you will experience new vitality and return to health... in *body and soul!*

David Hazard
Founder of The New Nature Institute

1

When Life Is a Vicious Cycle

*P*MS is the subject of a lot of jokes. Men tease women about it. Women offer up the latest definition ("pass my shotgun," "pardon my sobbing"), and late-night talk-show hosts never miss a chance to score a laugh with some new take on the malady. (What's the difference between a woman with PMS and a cow with Mad Cow Disease?—Lipstick.)

But for women who suffer from premenstrual syndrome, this condition is anything but a joke. If you suffer from PMS, you know that when it strikes, life can be an unhappy, uncomfortable ride.

First there are the monthly rounds of physical distress—everything from cramps, nausea, and bloating, to blood pressure fluctuations, headaches, and migraines. Then there's the emotional distress of mood swings. You can feel on top one minute...and an hour later struggle with depression or terrible anxiety. Along with that you may also experience mental distress: You feel irritable for no reason...and then you feel guilty for being irritable. You feel frustrated...but indecisive...and you wonder, "Am I just losing my mind?"

And on another level, there is the even greater toll PMS takes over time. After years of such distress you can sink mentally, emotionally, and spiritually under the heavy sense that PMS is limiting you...and you're missing out on so much of your own life.

Over time, many women who suffer from PMS can find themselves waging a battle with body, mind, and emotions—a battle that sometimes even brings them to the edge of despair. They wonder, "What kind of life could I be living...whose life could I be contributing to…what creative goals could I be reaching…if only *my* life wasn't caught in this vicious cycle?"

For such women, I have great news.

You can do something to remedy the distress caused by PMS. There are many natural strategies you can use to relieve and even conquer your worst symptoms. These natural remedies are safe, easy to use, and readily available to every woman who wants to escape the vicious cycle of PMS. (In fact, these strategies can bring welcome relief to *any* woman who suffers from distressing symptoms during her monthly cycle—even women who have not been "officially" diagnosed with PMS.)

Self-knowledge is always the first step in overcoming any personal problem. For that reason, it's important to know exactly what's going on inside your body during your monthly cycle. Then you can begin to find the best solutions.

What PMS Does to You

Conventional wisdom says women are more "in tune" with their bodies than men simply because they have to be. After all, once menstruation begins, they experience hormonal fluctuations and obvious physical symptoms. Because these changes happen roughly every 28 days like clockwork, a woman is *made* to focus on her body and know how it works.

Too often, it's thought that a woman *should* know her body. And so she *should* know what's wrong with her when she's suffering from PMS…just because she's a woman. This guilt-inducing idea only adds to her distress.

Stacey

Stacey had been athletic in high school and college, and she felt she had a good knowledge of her body. But in her mid-twenties, after her first child was born, she began experiencing severe headaches regularly. Her family physician told her it was probably the stress of a new marriage, new career, and new baby. In a well-meaning way, he patted her arm and gave offered this advice. "You're probably just a 'type-A' personality. Stop burning the candle at both ends, and I'll bet your headaches will stop."

He never associated her symptoms with PMS—though it's common for hormonal changes during a woman's cycle to trigger headaches and even migraines in some women.

If Stacey hadn't set out to find help for herself, had she not found natural remedies to treat her problem, she would still be suffering those excruciating monthly headaches.

Pat

Food was a real enemy in Pat's life. She didn't have an eating disorder—but half of the time food was mildly unappealing and she barely ate anything...while the other half of the time she was starving and ate ravenously.

As a result, her blood sugar fluctuated wildly. One week she was fatigued and dragging. The next she felt energetic—but then overate. Her size-6 clothes were now jammed into the back of her closet...while larger and larger sizes took their place. More importantly, as her weight rose, her desire to stay active decreased. She felt tired, tight, and like she'd begun to age almost overnight.

Fortunately, her gynecologist recognized that there was a definite pattern in her under- and overeating. As they discussed the pattern in detail, he was able to link it to hormonal fluctuations in her monthly cycle. Had her doctor missed this detail, Pat would never have sought the right solution to her problem.

Once she adopted a plan that included simple dietary adjustments, along with natural supplements, and the right program of mental, spiritual, and physical strategies to keep her energy level more constant throughout the month, her condition improved.

It's a myth, that every woman *should* automatically know what's going on in her body...just because she's a woman. If no one has described to you the process your body goes through, how *could* you know about the many chemical changes that go on invisibly inside you, often causing havoc through your whole being?

Now it's true that you may know very well what's going on with your body *symptomatically*—that is, you're well aware that you're experiencing cramps or moodswings. But has anyone really taken the time to help you understand your *hormonal cycle?* What hormones are released and when? How do they affect your brain, your central nervous system, your heart and blood vessels, and of course, your reproductive system?

Do you really know what incredible changes happen in your body from week to week for as long as you are menstruating?

DO YOU KNOW ABOUT PMDD ?

You know about PMS, and how severe it can be. But most women have never even heard of its more serious version—Premenstrual Dysmorphic Disorder, or PMDD.

Although some 50 percent of menstruating women experience PMS, only 3 to 5 percent experience PMDD.

The symptoms of PMDD are far more painful and severe than PMS. Women suffering from PMDD will experience heightened pain, more intense cramps, more gastrointestinal bloating, and worse headaches.

Most especially, women suffering from PMDD will experience more intense mood swings—making life an even more unbearable, unpredictable roller coaster of sadness, depression, irritability, and anxiety. Sometimes, women with PMDD can even become argumentative and aggressive, clashing with family and coworkers, and exploding in angry outbursts.

If you think that you or someone you know may be experiencing PMDD, consult a doctor for diagnosis and treatment. Although some natural remedies may help relieve the distress of PMDD, treatment with pharmaceutical medications may be necessary.

For some women the steps of the cycle, as explained in the following, will not be new information. Possibly your mother, older sister, or health teacher told you what was going on in your body during your monthly cycle. But even if you are well-informed, it will benefit you to review the various hormonal fluctuations that cause you distress.

Here is what your body is up to…and what its cyclical changes do to you.

The Vicious Cycle

First Week

During the first week of your cycle, you are menstruating. The uterine lining from your previous cycle has matured and is now being shed. This allows the new lining that's been forming underneath to take its place. The shedding period lasts about five days.

At the end of that time your body begins to produce more of several hormones.

One is estrogen. This hormone encourages your uterine lining to thicken, creating a soft "bed" inside your body to catch and nourish a fertilized egg.

☛ *This hormonal change is responsible for the cramping many women experience during the first part of their cycle.*

At the same time, the pituitary gland in your brain is increasing the production of other hormones. They travel to your ovaries… causing eggs to begin maturing. Several will actually begin the process (though normally only one grows fastest and is soon released).

☛ *These additional hormonal fluctuations are responsible for mood swings and increased appetite during this time.*

Second Week

All those eggs developing inside your ovaries produce more estrogen and also progesterone. This is the week when estrogen reaches its greatest level in your cycle.

At the end of this week, somewhere around the fourteenth day, the follicle that is most-developed releases its egg. When the egg is released, you may feel a slight "twinge" in your pelvis.

☛ *For many women, this week is "free space"—the time in their cycle when they experience few symptoms or none at all. Some feel energized, productive, creative, more "balanced."*

Third Week

Now the egg is making its way down one of your fallopian tubes. The follicle that launched it is producing more progesterone.

Progesterone causes blood vessels to swell, which helps the uterine lining thicken a bit more in anticipation of a possible pregnancy. This directs more blood-borne nutrients to your uterus. They'll be needed if the egg becomes fertilized and implants itself in your uterine wall.

☛ *Because of all the energy and activity being directed to your uterus, you are likely to experience bloating and more cramps this third week. You may also experience breast tenderness. As a result of slightly increased blood pressure, you may also suffer from irritability and anxiety.*

☛ *Additionally, because the blood vessels are expanding, women who are prone to chronic headaches and migraines may experience them during this week.*

Fourth Week

If your egg is fertilized—**Congratulations! You're going to be a mom!** You've won a pass to get off the cycle for about a year.

But if your egg is not fertilized it rapidly disintegrates, and it will be flushed out of your body with the flow that begins next week.

Progesterone production drops rapidly. Your blood vessels slowly return to normal.

☛ *Unfortunately, many of the unpleasant symptoms from last week are likely to continue into this week—including cramps, breast tenderness, headaches...and that hard-to-manage anxiety and moodiness.*

Next week the cycle starts up again, and you get to go through it all over...and over...and over. That is, unless you implement a way to balance out those wild hormonal and vascular changes that make your life the wild ride it is.

℞

YOUR BEST BET IS A TEAM APPROACH

~

Here are two thoughts about building a supportive team to help you control PMS.

1. It's important to work with knowledgeable healthcare professionals. You are likely to benefit from blood- and other diagnostic tests that can pinpoint problem areas...and from the knowledge of doctors, nutritionists, naturopaths, and others in the broader spectrum of healthcare.

The information offered in this book is meant to supplement, not replace their advice.

2. If you're resistant to developing a relationship with healthcare professionals, you can work to get beyond it.

Here are some of the common reasons women give for not getting good healthcare attention:

- "A doctor told me he didn't believe me when I told him about my symptoms. He said it was all in my head and that I was exaggerating."

- "My mother and grandmother taught me just to tough it out."

- "Healthcare is expensive, and money's tight."

- "I'm embarrassed to be examined."

- "My children come first. They see the doctor, but I rarely do."

- "I had a very bad experience with a doctor, and I can't bring myself to go back."

Even though there are effective natural remedies you can use, there is no reason good enough for not finding the right healthcare professionals to help in your efforts to control PMS...or any other ailment you are suffering.

Make the commitment today to take better care of yourself.

Fortunately, there are indeed ways to restore well-being in body, mind, and spirit...naturally.

Creating a Strategy for Taming PMS— One that Works for You

There was a reason for breaking down your monthly cycle into its weekly components. Knowing *what* changes are going on inside you and *when* can help you determine which natural remedies to use at the proper time.

In fact, the strategies that fill the balance of this book will help you in two important ways.

1. **You will be able to create a personal strategy that supports your own "core sense of well-being."**

   Some of the strategies support a balanced sense of overall wellness in body, mind, and spirit. They'll help you maintain inner balance, serenity, and a sense of well-being that extends throughout your whole cycle. These are strategies you will want to use on a daily basis, to create a strong core of healthy vitality in body, mind, and spirit.

2. **You will be able to create a troubleshooting plan—one that relieves those PMS symptoms that are specifically distressing you.**

   Many of the remedies in this book work naturally and effectively to prevent or relieve cramps, bloating, muscle aches, headaches and migraines, hormonal fluctuations, mood swings, and other symptoms of PMS. These are the strategies you will want to use to target symptoms you normally experience during the various weeks of your cycle.

   Best of all, you will be able to develop a plan that treats you like a whole person—taking into account the needs of body, mind, and spirit.

If you want to create a personal plan that helps make your life manageable again, read each of the following chapters carefully. You'll want to test the strategies suggested to see which ones work for you. In this way, you can develop a plan that fits your specific needs.

This will mean creating the two-track approach mentioned previously, using strategies that give you both a "core of well-being" and the ability to "troubleshoot," counteracting distressing symptoms as they occur.

Whether you've suffered from premenstrual syndrome for a long time or the distress is fairly new, you can learn to control PMS...*naturally*.

2

Cleansing Your Mind

Our state of mind has a powerful effect on our well-being. To see just how true that is, put yourself in this scenario.

You come home at noontime and check your phone messages. The first one's a hang-up, but the second call is from someone close. Let's say it's one of your children or an elderly parent...sounding a bit anxious. "Call me right away. It's urgent." You feel slightly alarmed.

But you call back, and there's no answer. You call around and can't find them.

An hour goes by...and then the whole afternoon. Your concern turns to worry. What was the emergency? Are they in a hospital somewhere right now, sick or injured? You shoot up little prayers. Please let them call...please let them be okay....

By evening...still no word. You have a slight headache behind your eyes, and your stomach feels knotted. You're not really hungry and only pick at dinner.

Night comes, and you turn off the late news—which was supposed to distract, but has made you more anxious. Too many terrible things happening out there, and every story has wrung on your emotions. Now your prayers have an impatient, even angry, edge. Why aren't you helping, God? I need to hear something....

Finally! The phone rings. "Sorry if I scared you," comes the explanation. "But I was going out for the whole day, and I was just calling about the family picnic. I said it was urgent because I thought I might get to the grocery store, and I wanted to know before I left what kind of food you want me to bring...."

The relief you feel hopefully balances out the anger—about the whole day you just spent in a really unpleasant state of mind.

Have you ever experienced something like this? Can you relate to it? As the previous scenario shows, an agitated state of mind can have a powerful negative impact—not just on our mental well-being, but on our physical and spiritual well-being, too.

Fortunately, the opposite is also true. A calm, relaxed state of mind has a positive impact on every aspect of our being. As many women have discovered, a balanced and serene state of mind—a mind cleansed of stress, anxiety, and negativity—is one of the most powerful allies in controlling PMS.

The Healing Power of a Sound Mind

Listen to what these women have to say about the health-supporting powers of the mind.

> When the PMS symptoms started up every month I'd immediately feel sorry for myself. I'd think, *My husband doesn't understand. My boss doesn't know or care.*...I honestly had no idea how this mind-set was building up to one big case of depression. And I definitely had no clue how that made my physical condition even worse.
>
> Then I learned a little technique that taught me how to step back from myself. That helped me see how I was letting my mood control my thoughts and my body. I learned how to take control of my mind. That's when I turned the corner with this PMS thing. The change was dramatic.
>
> —*Sharon N.*

> I learned that you can create a healthy state of mind...a deep state of serenity inside. I could feel my soul relaxing. Once I knew how to do that, I wasn't *under* the pain anymore. I was able to get *above* it, so to speak. It's gotten so I actually

have a pretty good degree of control over the headaches and cramps and actually help them ease away.

—*Geraldine B.*

Every month I had these wild mood swings. I'd be sweet to my kids one minute, and screaming at them the next. I'd be awful to my husband—he never knew what he was getting when he walked in the door. I'd hate myself, and think, *What a horrible wife and mother. What a witch.* But I learned I didn't have to be this big "victim" of my own moods.

I started using some simple mental strategies—they were actually pretty easy to learn—and very quickly I could *even out* my emotions. It was amazing. No more roller coaster. My husband and kids will tell you…what a huge change! I don't hate myself every month.

—*Nanci G.*

An ancient text from the Bible refers to the interior strength— a "power" that brings us to wholeness—that comes from "a sound mind."[1] By that, the biblical writer meant "a self-disciplined" mind.[2] We might also think of it as a *self-cleansing* mind—one that knows how to cleanse itself of the stresses and junk of life that pass through it every day.

Each of the women who shared their thoughts above demonstrates the healing power of a disciplined mind in dealing with PMS.

Sharon learned to "step back" and recognize that hormonally induced moods compounded her mental misery. When she saw the problem, she turned to a healthier mental strategy and did something to relieve the anguish in her mind.

Geraldine learned how to use her mind to create a serene state, indirectly bringing peace to her spirit. (We'll look at techniques that directly influence the spirit in the next chapter.) In short, Geraldine learned how to create the mental state known as "flow." Medical researchers know that "flow-thinking" triggers the body's relaxation response—that is, a deeply at-rest state of mind, body, and spirit that actually causes the body to release healing and pain-relieving hormones. That relaxation response helped Geraldine experience real physical changes and relief from her PMS symptoms.

Nanci used some mental techniques to even out her moods. She learned that it's possible—even if you experience states of high anxiety or agitation—to smooth out the rough emotional ride going on inside you. And so she was able to escape her emotional roller coaster and become more in charge of herself again, more calm and even-tempered.

To have a disciplined mind does not mean to become brainy, or studious, or bookish. It doesn't mean buying into New Age claims that the mind has "fantastic powers that can change reality."

Rather, a disciplined mind uses widely recognized mental strategies to cleanse your head of

- stress-inducing thoughts
- emotionally charged thoughts
- general negativity

—all of which contribute to poor health in general, and also amplify the symptoms of specific physical conditions like PMS.

So…what are the mental strategies you can use to control the effects of PMS? You'll want to try each of these out for yourself and find out how to make them work for you.

The Mental Strategies

Strategy #1: Mind-Body Breathing

(Use this anywhere for simple, quick stress release.)

Women who suffer from PMS feel especially bombarded from all sides. Moods zoom up and down like the stock market on a bad day. Mentally, you feel distracted, sluggish, or unclear. Add to that several demands on you at once—a ringing phone, kids needing your attention, office or housework to do—and you've got that "shakey inside" feeling that warns you you're on *stress overload*.

Unfortunately, stress overload can hit you anywhere. In a meeting at the office. Dealing with a child. In a checkout line at the store. Suddenly you feel the "adult" part of you unravel…and the angry you—or the upset and teary you—comes out. It's not pretty. Instead of letting stress build till it rattles you apart again…

Do This:

1. Call a mental time-out.

Instead of taking charge right now, try letting go. Take a moment to tell yourself, "Wait a minute. Right at the moment, this is all too much for me. I need a breather."

2. Take a breather—literally.

Take a deep breath. Let it in slowly through your nose, filling your chest, feeling your diaphragm expand…and let it out quickly through your mouth. Hear yourself make a quiet "huffing" noise like you'd make if you were cleaning your glasses lens. (More on the physical benefits of doing this in a later chapter.)

3. Puff the stress out.

Take another deep breath…in and out…rolling your shoulders to stretch and release any tension that's gathered there.

Repeat…letting your ribs expand…focusing on releasing stress there.

Again…letting the intake of air cause your diaphragm and lower abdomen fill—the way a baby's tummy rises when she breathes—and focus on releasing stress caught in your midsection.

4. See the stress go. Hear peace return.

Just refocusing your mind off the external pressures and onto your breathing may be enough to restore mental calm. An additional step may help:

- In your mind's eye, picture the stress as an object—a feather or a mist—that you are blowing away from you with each exhale.

- As you let go of stress with each breath, repeat a positive affirmation. You can use a physical command or go soul-deep with a soothing scripture:

"My mind is calm."

"My body is relaxed. The stress is leaving. I'm peaceful now."

"I have 'the peace of God that is beyond understanding.'"

"Peace…be still."

- Listen for that "still small voice" to speak calming words within.

Strategy #2: Mindkeeping

Use this when the mental clutter of "too many details" is stressing you.

Okay, so maybe you've never been the most organized person. Or maybe you're normally on top of things except when PMS is frying your circuits.

In either case, here's what happens in your head: You take stock of what you have to accomplish today or this week. You begin to make mental lists of all the details for each task that needs to be done. Subliminally, your stress level is rising. Respiration gets shallow (which is why you need the first strategy). Stress hormones are released, and blood pressure rises (which is why you need this one, too.) Without realizing it you've induced a state of stressful thinking.

When this happens, you are *overwhelmed.* Suddenly, you can't think straight. Your ability to order things and set priorities temporarily vanishes…and you don't know where to begin. All the important, must-get-done details of your life are shuffled like so many notecards with commands scribbled on them. Emotionally, you feel defeated as you watch the puzzle pieces that are your day or week get strewn in chaos on the floor. You feel overwhelmed. Defeated.

Some women try checking out. Letting the house go. Dropping out of activities. But taking this route can have negative repercussions. Maybe it's not even an option.

If PMS regularly messes up the "inner house" of your mind, you can benefit from these "mindkeeping" techniques. (This strategy begins with a familiar technique...but adds a twist to give you better coping power.)

Do This:

1. Set aside one part of a day each month for "executive planning."

You *are* the CEO of your life, whether you realize it or not. Executives need time to give order to the demands on them. Choose a morning, afternoon, or evening. Just make a regular space in your month, and try not to violate it. During this time, you will

- *Anchor important dates on your calendar* (like meetings, necessary home and auto maintenance, kids' events, shopping trips). Note which days are going to be most demanding.

- *Schedule a period of rest before every difficult day.* You can't predict all the rough days...but some of them you can. And to get through them without being overwhelmed, you need to realize the wisdom of pacing yourself. The day before your demanding days...give yourself an afternoon or evening "off" to rest, breathe deep, relax, and prepare.

2. Take an hour each weekend to "rough in" your week on a pocket planner.

Here's where it's handy to own a small planner you can tuck in your purse or briefcase. You may want to use one that shows you only a week at a time—especially if you can't help looking ahead to next week and borrowing stress from the future (a bad habit many of us do).

- *Write down the important anchoring events. And those important break times.* This will reinforce your need for breaks and keep you from "cheating" by letting them fill in with spur-of-the-moment demands.

- *List other needs, demands, and invitations that have come up. Pre-sort your list.* Before you write anything more on your weekly planner, go through your list of upcomings events and choose: Which are *most* important...which can you let go. An enormous amount of mental stress comes from being weak in the ability to say *yes* and *no.* Many women erode their mental, physical, and spiritual health because they're afraid of not looking like super woman or of letting someone down.

  Learn when to say *yes*...and when to say *no.* Accept your human limitations. Delegate where you can. Issue apologies where necessary.

- *Plan to accomplish three, no more than four, of the things on your "important" list in any given week. Schedule no more than one thing from your "important" list on any given day.* Does this sound like an effort to help you simplify your life? It is. Stress is the number one killer of adults. We all need to dial-down the pressure.

  But you're thinking, *How will I get everything done?* The fact is you still have the demands of everyday life to get through. And other, small, spontaneous demands will tend to spring up—they always do. That's the point of leaving spaces in your plans—unexpected demands on your time drift in, the way hollows fill up with falling snow.

3. Each morning, jot down a To Do List.

You've got your priorities scheduled. You've got your agenda. Now let's account for the wild cards that might get dealt to you today.

- *Handling the "snowdrift" of spontaneous demands.* "Could you just"—don't you hate the word *just?*—"write up these meeting minutes," "pick up my dry cleaning," "buy me school supplies?" Everyone around is trying to get you to do their agenda. What you may need is...

some personal esteem. Don't let guilt erode the balance you're working for. You are not a "bad" mother, wife, daughter, sister, or friend if you can't meet everyone's needs and demands. Remind yourself it's all right to be human and have limits.

a good "script." Don't know how to speak up for your needs? Here are some suggestions: "My schedule is so full, I just can't get to that today." Or "Today is a busy one for me, and I'm also not feeling well physically." Or, if you really want to be generous: "I won't promise anything because I have important things to get done—but if I have energy and time left at the end of the day I'll see if I can fit it in."

• *Prepare for the unexpected, and for delays.* Everything usually takes longer than we expect. Life is made up of delays, delays, delays. We *know* this—so let's *plan* for it. How?

Add 30 to 45 minutes to the time allotted for *each thing* you plan to do in a given day. You'll be surprised to find that this alone keeps your schedule just about on target!

Draw a line across your daily To Do List to divide the list in half. Many women plan more for a given day than they can handle. When PMS is already causing distress, it only adds to your mental pressure and emotional depression to look at a To Do List late in the day and see that it's still half full. Your mental state will cause you to focus on what you *haven't* accomplished instead of on what you *have.*

Drawing a line at the halfway point across your list has these benefits: First, it's probably a lot more realistic list of what you can really get done. (Remember this and adjust your future schedules accordingly!) Second, there is something mentally and emotionally relaxing about crossing any finish line. Anything you do beyond the halfway line puts you mentally in the bonus category, leaving you with a positive sense about yourself.

4. Affirm yourself at the end of the day...for what you accomplished and for what you wisely said no to.

As an adult woman—who affirms you? Affirmation is rare for *every* adult. We have to do this for ourselves. It's how we build a healthy self-assessment.

Look over your To Do List and tell yourself: "I got *this, this,* and *this* done—and that was good. And I didn't take on *that* unnecessary pressure—that was good, too. And what I didn't accomplish, I can reschedule."

For any woman who has struggled with disorganization, this strategy offers many obvious benefits. For the woman with PMS—who is already struggling for mental clarity and emotional balance—this mindkeeping strategy can reduce mental stress and it's side-effects of emotional distress, relational tensions, and physical discomforts.

Strategy #3: Cleansing Your Thought-flow

For handling emotionally charged thoughts that trigger those awful ups and downs.

Being hormonal and being emotional go hand in hand. The hormones flow, and moods swing—sometimes from hour to hour. With PMS, the effects are even more exaggerated. The highs (when there are any) are higher and the lows are...*watch out.* We're talking "chasm" here!

Moods are like tributaries of our consciousness. Think of your moods as one current, pouring into the river of your running thoughts. Here's how it works.

Last week, when you felt okay, someone made a mildly negative comment about your appearance. In response, you had a neutral thought—based in logic: "That was rude." Or "I think I look okay. What's their problem?" It was easier to let the comment go.

This week, with hormones giving you a rough go, you hear the same mildly negative comment. Whatever emotion is flowing in at the moment—anxiety, insecurity, sadness, or angry agitation—*flows into* the stream of your logic. In fact, it pretty well drowns out all logic.

Reason, your great defender, is overwhelmed. Now your thoughts are emotionally charged, and this gives them enormous power...over *you*.

So what happens?

The comment goes straight to heart. You feel deeply wounded, put down, and rejected. Self-image is part of our identity...and yours just took a big hit. Even if you counter with an angry, defensive response ("Oh yeah? Well just look at the size of your *thighs*"), underneath it all you *still* feel defeated at a basic level of your being.

To make it worse, because your hormones keep the emotional stream pouring in, your thoughts *stay* emotionally charged for a long time after. You replay the insult all day. (It's not that you're nasty and unforgiving—*you're hormonal!*) And this amplifies the emotion in your mind.

Maybe this *isn't* you. But if it is...

Do This:

1. During your most emotional times...spend some time alone and identify the emotions running through your head.

Most people have a dominant set of emotions. Yours may be in the sad spectrum ("blue," unhappiness, sense of grief). Or the agitated spectrum (irritable, annoyed, quick-tempered). Or on the fearful side (nervous, anxious, near panic). Or even the dark end of emotions (loss of caring, depression, despair).

Because we're human, we're capable of having different emotions and even conflicting emotions at the same time. But we will normally have a dominant set. (Note: Conflicting emotions may *be* your dominant set. If you find yourself "hung up" and indecisive a lot, this is likely the case.)

Sitting or walking by yourself, focus in on the emotional stream going on inside you.

2. Watch how the emotions mix with your logical thoughts...to form a new thought.

Emotionally charged thoughts are usually the ones that have a negative impact on your balance and well-being. Watching how they change and color your thoughts is something like watching food coloring swirl into a cake batter. You really can perceive their effects on you if you try. So,

- *Observe your mood-flow and verbalize it to yourself.* ("I've been anxious all morning.")

- *Observe the topic(s) you're thinking about.* (Job. Home. Relationships. Health. Appearance.) When we're in balance, our thoughts on any topic tend to be neutral and factual. ("I haven't called my best friend in a while." "My workload is heavy, and I'm not getting it all done.")

- *Observe how your mood is pulling your logical thinking into its current.* ("I'm so worried that I've neglected [a friend], and I've probably hurt her." "I'm anxious because this job is getting beyond me, and I'll never catch up—in fact, my boss is probably thinking about firing me right now.")

- *Observe how turning up the reason-flow soothes the mood-flow.* When emotions are wildly out of control, you need a simpler strategy—such as the first strategy in this chapter—mind-body breathing. But when you've gotten some internal control, you *do* need to deal with your thought-flow. Talking logically to your emotions will turn down the mental stress they cause.

We're not talking about giving yourself a "stern talking to" or "moralizing" at yourself ("I shouldn't feel this way." *Why not?—You're human aren't you?*) We're talking about simply stating facts...mentioning objective steps you can take. ("I'll call my friend and apologize for neglecting her." "I'll talk to my boss and ask for help in creating a strategy so the work will get done. That way I won't look negligent, but thoughtful and responsible."

Yes, you can take charge of emotionally charged thoughts. If you use this strategy, it will help keep you from feeling like you're losing it or going crazy during those difficult times of your cycle.

(A final tip: You can also adapt this strategy for use in conversations that derail because emotions get charged up—and watch the dynamics of your relationships change for the better!)

Strategy #4: Get Out of Your Head

(This simple practice works like a small miracle...in just minutes.)

Sometimes stress and emotions and mental overload are just...there. The day's schedule is shot and you'd shred your pocket planner...if you could find it. Emotionally charged thoughts, fueled by your hormones, are dragging you around by the heart. And now you don't have enough energy to do much about it.

When mental stress and emotional overload are overwhelming you, and all else fails...

Do This:

1. If possible, step out of your immediate circumstances.

Excuse yourself from the meeting for a moment...leave the grocery cart...take a break from the stressful conversation...pull the car over.

Changing your setting—even if you take just a few steps away from where you were—adds to the sense of leaving your mental stress behind. If you can't leave the location you're in, proceed with the following steps....

2. Focus your eyes intently on a fixed spot anywhere from one to three feet ahead of you.

When we're tense, every part of our being tends to bear down. Muscles tense. Eyes zoom in intently on The Problem. We fix our gaze at a point that's very close—from one to three feet in front us—"boring a hole into it" with our eyes.

Notice that you are most likely looking down. Feel the stress in your body, your face, your forehead, and your eyes.

3. Let your eyes drift upward...let your focus broaden... until you are staring into the distance.

We can actually reverse our feelings of stress and intensity by refocusing our gaze. Letting our eyes drift up—until they come to rest in the blue sky above the horizon—or at a blank spot high on the wall—triggers a relaxation response that spreads from the top of our head down through our body.

Notice that you automatically draw a cleansing breath. Allow yourself to keep breathing deeply. Feel how the release of muscle tension reestablishes mental calm, emotional balance, and even a sense of physical well-being.

By letting this quick strategy work its small miracle you can re-enter the situation you stepped away from and not allow PMS to rob you of your serenity and that in-charge feeling you need.

3

Empowering Your Spirit

"A bright spirit…gives health…."[3]

Believe it or not, you carry with you, every day—even on the days when PMS has you feeling your worst—one of the most powerful sources of health and well-being in existence. That tremendous source of wellness is your *spirit*.

Until recently, the medical community has been skeptical and even dismissive of the role that the human spirit plays in healing and overall wellness. But the evidence is in. Many studies have shown that patients with painful, "incurable" illnesses—even patients judged "terminal"—have come back to health and made full recoveries. How?

Most people who made remarkable recoveries claim it was by discovering that they could create conditions deep inside themselves that "allowed" health and well-being to return. As a woman named Jamie puts it:

> I became aware that I had allowed the way I was living—not outwardly so much as inside—to become very unhealthy. For one thing, I was carrying a lot of deep-level tension, because I was living in opposition to some of my most important values. For another, I was way out-of-line with what I wanted to do vocationally with my life.
>
> At the time I discovered this, a spiritual man I know offered me advice. He listened, and he understood my problem. He helped me see that I hadn't practiced good spiritual habits. And so I'd allowed the unhealthy conditions inside me to grow over time. He helped me to not feel guilty or stupid that I'd allowed this to happen, by pointing out that I just hadn't known before how to maintain good

spiritual health. Then he introduced me to certain spiritual practices that were very "doctoring" for my spirit. They've helped me create new, healthier conditions deep inside.

I've suffered from PMS symptoms [and another chronic illness] ever since I was a teenager. But since I started using these spiritual practices, the pain and discomfort [of PMS] has dropped dramatically. And the mood swings…well, I've really learned how to take charge and minimize them. I feel good now. I like myself and my life again.

You Are Not a Body that Owns a Spirit, You Are a Spirit Who Lives in a Body

Within you, there burns a flame. Not an ordinary flame because it can't be seen by the human eye nor will it never go out. This flame is your living spirit…the life deep within you. It vitalizes your body and whispers to your beleaguered, distracted mind about the deeply important matters of life. It's the part of you that was ignited and breathed into you by the Maker of every living thing.[4]

In the Bible, the psalmist referred to this eternal part of every person as their "inmost being."[5] The Hebrew word that is translated as "inmost being" actually means…your deepest, most important values, hopes, and dreams; your very personhood. It's the person who's *really* in there when everyone else's demands and expectations are peeled away…the essential, core *you*. If your spirit is strong and well, the Bible tells us, it will give us a vitality that radiates from the center of our body into our very bones.[6]

Today, even the healthcare community—which once viewed us as a collection of chemicals and matter—is recognizing that the human spirit is real and potent. It isn't just some filmy wisp of ourselves that trots out to ooh and ah at inspiring sunsets, or the urge we feel to do charity work or go to worship. More healthcare practitioners than ever before are convinced that we are not mere bio-mechanical machines, and that our core self—our "inmost being"—has a powerful part in determining the state of our health and well-being.

What the doctors of both spirit *and* body now agree on is this:

If your spirit is unhealthy—weak, worn down, out of balance—it can contribute to poor health. Opportunistic illnesses and weaknesses in your physical being win the day you become ill, and your pain is amplified. But if your spirit is well—if it's in a healthy state—it has a big role in supporting your well-being and minimizing pain throughout your body.

Even if you suffer from the worst PMS symptoms, creating a healthy spirit will help you experience more well-being and freedom from discomfort. The key, as Jamie and many other women are discovering, lies in using spiritual practices—many of them known to Christians for millennia before us—that lead to health that wells up from deep within and balances your whole being.

You too can learn to use these spiritual practices—or strategies—to remedy PMS symptoms. As with all spiritual practices, of course, they'll benefit more than your body. You can expect them to help you grow in your relationship with God and with other people as well.

What follows are strategies that will empower your spirit. By testing them all, you'll find the ones most helpful in relieving your particular distress.

The Spiritual Practices
Strategy #1: Start a New Dance with God

The way we relate to God is a central issue in each of our lives. Also, just as important is what we think *God thinks* about us. If we're in tension with a Being who is absolutely central in our lives, we will carry a core-level stress all the time. And stress at this level can show up in symptoms in our physical bodies—from suppressed immune and hormonal functioning to hypertension and high blood pressure—and in our mental and emotional state as well—from depression, cynicism, and bitterness about life, to mood swings.

Learning how to have a healthy, balanced relationship with God is actually a matter that's central to our total health and well-being.

Many people of faith believe they have a good relationship with God. But going by the vast number of people seeking pastoral and therapeutic help with major life issues, it seems we have *a lot* of what are often called "God issues." We want to be close to God—but then stuff happens. We do things that seem wrong. Things happen to us that are hurtful or bad. Suddenly we're not so sure about this God-relationship we're trying to have. As a result...

Every one of us does a dance with God. This dance has a name—it's called, "Today, I'll Move Close to You, Tomorrow I'll Move Away." Here are two variations:

Variation #1: One day you're feeling pretty good about yourself—the things you say and do, the way you see yourself treating people. On those days, you're pretty sure God is happy to be around you. You move close to God and feel confident about praying, confiding, asking for things. You feel God understands and likes you.

Then...let's say PMS strikes. You feel rotten and stressed, and you hear yourself being snappish, impatient, even mean...or just see yourself "not there" for those who need you.

Now you're pretty sure God is not happy with you. After all, God is one who says things like, "Love your neighbor as yourself." Because you've violated that rule—how could God be happy with you...much less want to be around you, crabby as you are?

As a result, you feel guilt and ashamed...and you "dance" away from God. And in the silent space that opens up, you imagine God's cosmic disappointment or anger and wonder just *how* disgusted God really is with you anyway.

Variation #2: Sometimes your life is good. Maybe not great... just manageable, but you'll take it. Or maybe your life is bringing you some nice "bennies" and perks—even better.

In your dance with God, you feel as if God has moved close, and you whisper things like, "This is good. Just keep it this way."

Then something sad or painful happens. You feel like you've been punched in the soul. How did this happen? Where did God go? You feel like God suddenly backed off and left you dancing without a partner. What's up with this cosmic disappearing act? And even more important—how can you trust yourself to dance with God again if God is going to let bad things sneak up and suddenly knock the wind out of your soul? Isn't it God's job to love and protect you?

So, in your dance with God you back off a few steps. If the blow you felt was bad enough, you may even decide to "sit it out" with this faith business. Forget praying. And *really* forget worship. If God wants to show up and make good, your phone number and address are in the book.

What you need to recognize is that your idea of "dancing with God" is based on *conditions*. One set of conditions is *your behavior*—you believe God comes close or backs off depending on how you act. The other set of conditions is *God's behavior*—you believe that when life is good God is good, and when life is bad God are bad.

With this mindset, someone is always under judgment—either yourself or God. And a spirit full of judgment is a life-drainer. (Can you see why Jesus said, "Do not judge"? [7])

It's time to start a new dance with God.

Do This:

1. Stop setting conditions on whether you will or will not stay in the "dance" with God. Step in the dance, and stay in.

Every one of us sets unspoken conditions on whether we'll step away from God or step closer to Him.

When we judge ourselves to be bad, we let guilt and shame cause us to step away from God. When bad things happen we let our disappointment and anger cause us to step away, too.

We stop basing our dance with God on the conditions we set when we say, "I will stay in this with you, God—unconditionally. I want to grow in a more mature, healthy, and stable relationship with you—whatever that means."

2. Be willing to follow God's lead. Be willing to have your eyes opened to God's way of seeing and doing things.

☞ *In our personal life*

From our perspective, if someone blows it—that may be *it*. Sure, we'll give certain favored people a bunch of chances. There must, however, be a limit. But that's our way of seeing things.

Christianity teaches that when we blow it we can always turn to God and find grace and forgiveness. "God is love," the Bible teaches—but many of us have had our spirit toxified by an opposite message: "God loves you *if...*" And we never meet all the conditions of that *if*, do we?

God *is* love. And from God's perspective, our failures are opportunities to learn and grow.

We need to stop backing off *from God* after we've failed, and instead move closer *to God*. Only in this way can we experience welcome and forgiveness...and only in this way can we begin to correct our real missteps and failings.

☞ *In the big issues of life*

From our perspective, life has fair and unfair aspects. Because God is supposedly in charge of running this universe, God must be fair sometimes...and unfair sometimes. (Back to that judging thing again.)

Christianity also teaches (as do most other religious traditions, by the way) that God is not a cosmic Merchant in the Marketplace, measuring out beans in a balance. God is not Santa Claus, checking his list to see who gets rewarded with better presents...and who gets coal.

Hebrew-Christian wisdom tells us that God's ways are higher than our ways. Sometimes we're allowed to experience very difficult realities. These are no more punishments than the good things we experience are rewards. Jesus taught, in fact, that the rain "falls on the righteous and the unrighteous"[8] alike.

When we stop judging whether or not God is happy with us based on our limited view of tough realities that come our way, we begin to see—just a little bit—the way God sees.

3. Be willing to keep dancing until you understand the purpose of God's particular dance with you.

We do need to see where we've been wrong in our personal actions and we do need to see where we've been right. We also need to see where we've had right motives...but terrible methods.

Once we stop retreating from God into guilt and shame (or pride!) and begin to look at ourselves without the crippling effects of judgment, we start to see ourselves more honestly. If we accept that God is not disgusted with us...but guiding and directing us... we learn and grow.

Likewise, we do need to sense the purpose in our struggles with life. If we stop shutting God out in an effort to "punish" him for letting us down, if we keep asking to see our life from greater, wiser perspectives, we will gain insights about life and the human condition. We'll see that everyone suffers, and we're not alone or singled out for abuse by the universe.

It's then that an amazing transition takes place inside us. We start to gain an empowering grace, a compassion and ability to comfort and support other people who are struggling with life's tough issues. We'll eventually find there *is* purpose...and it may lie *especially* in our shared struggles.

This is God's long dance. And to stay in it we need to keep asking, "What do I need to know about life...and about other people...that I have yet to learn? Show me your greater purposes in our struggles."

If you make a practice of learning this new dance with God, you will find that your spirit becomes flexible and you are open to learning and growing. You'll experience a greater sense of God's love and patience...and a new vitality and excitement, coming from the closer relationship you're creating with God.

Strategy #2: Be Still...and Rest Your Spirit

Every time you turn around, someone is demanding something from you—right? Your husband or boyfriend, your family, your boss, your friends. Some days your schedule is overflowing, and then it gets interrupted…and then even your interruptions get interrupted.

On days when PMS symptoms are in gear it feels like life is eating you alive. You feel near tears…ready to scream. Thoughts are scattered. Your spirit feels agitated and anxious. You're being drained of any ounce of vitality you had. By the end of the day you feel stressed, exhausted, headachy, and sick.

Wouldn't it be great to be able to create a core sense of calm? To have an inner place of serenity where balance and control can be restored when the day's distractions are making you feel scattered and stressed to the max?

What you need is the simple practice of silent prayer…also known as *contemplative quiet*.

Learning this ancient Christian practice restores calm and order to scattered spirits, and also a sense that we are not overwhelmed by life but that we are once again in control.

And this practice has physical benefits, as well. When we experience deep-level calm, we trigger the deep-relaxation response. This releases hormones that boost our immune system and our mood. Physical resilience is restored. Women who practice this kind of prayer have reported that headaches ease, nausea and cramps subside, and energy returns. If this sounds great to you…

Do This:

1. Choose a quiet time…and a solitary place.

Pick the time when you're likely to be at your peak—able to be alert and focused. If you're going to practice this kind of praying it will take time though, so choose a spot in your schedule—or make one—that you can stick to.

As to place—you don't need a pristine wilderness, a church, or a monastery. All you need is a place where you can be *alone*. This can be a room in your home where no one will disturb you, a bench on your porch, a garden, or a park.

2. Clear your inner atmosphere.

This may take a little time, as there are several parts to it.

First, if something is bothering your conscience...admit it. Give your mistakes and failures over to God, and don't let them distract you now. (Keep yourself from going on guilt-trips. They never accomplish anything good—but they often further drain you spiritually.)

Second, take time to let your mind and spirit disentangle from the events of everyday life. You'll find yourself wanting to rehearse that unfinished conversation or worry over something you've left undone. (For this reason, keep a notepad with you to quickly jot down things you need to remember. This will allow you to relax again, knowing you'll remember to deal with them later.)

3. Focus on the stillness.

A simple start-up technique is to focus on your breathing. Close your eyes if it helps. Breathe in slowly through your nose... and release quickly through your mouth.

At first you'll be focused on the wave-like rhythm of your breath...the rise and fall of your ribs and abdomen. Eventually, you'll experience something else—a sense of *alertness*. When you become aware of the stillness behind any noise or motion...focus on the stillness.

4. Remain alert.

Some spiritual traditions emphasize just the emptying of interior space. In the Hebrew-Christian practice of contemplation, sweeping the house of the spirit clean is only a prelude to a wondrous event—a spiritual encounter with God.

No, you're not likely to hear an audible voice or see heavenly lights. You *are* likely to experience flashes of insight...and maybe even experience your physical symptoms abating.

(Be sure to write down any sense of insight you receive. Then spend time later considering whether or not it's helpful and valid.)

When your time of contemplative quiet is over you will simply feel your focus turning back out to normal, everyday things. But you will feel refreshed from deep within, with a freshness that flows from your spirit into your thoughts...and even into your body.

Strategy #3: Spiritual Journaling

Much of the stress we carry at a deep level comes from the fact that our spirit is carrying conflict—and maybe *many* conflicts. Sometimes we have misgivings, gut-feelings, vague longings, rest-lessness…a sense that we're missing something, but not sure what. These feelings are usually indications of conflicts that have settled deep within. Because your spirit is your core self—the essence of your life—the more conflicts you carry in your spirit and the bigger they are, the more you'll feel like you're disconnected from life.

When does this "life is out-of-sync" feeling and "the big dis-connect" show up most? You guessed it—on the days when you're least able to handle it…which is on those hormonal days, isn't it?

A "sense" or vague feeling is often like a tiny voice, shouting off in the distance, just beyond your hearing, trying to tell you that you are…

- living out of sync with a core value
- living without a greater sense of purpose
- living with conflicted perceptions about a person or situation

Unfortunately, most of us have so many superficial immediate demands, we don't take time to stop and listen to what our spirit is trying to tell us. Many women *almost* give in and listen when they're at their "PMS-iest"—but then the hormonal rage settles down and they ignore the voice of their spirit. Maybe they know that the voice would speak to them about making changes they're just afraid to make…. But as time goes on, conflicts in your spirit will only get worse unless you work to resolve them.

Journaling is a spiritual practice used for centuries, and it's a great way to listen to what your spirit is telling you. If you're in a growing relationship with God, it's a great way to hear what God may be whispering, too, in those silent, sacred spaces within. Many women, in fact, use contemplative quiet and journaling together. It makes for a satisfying combination of deep-spirit listening…fol-lowed by "giving voice" to still-unresolved questions and needs. And it's a wonderful way to capture and explore greater insights that come.

There are many reasons to journal—to capture memories of your family or love life, to record your ideas for creative projects. To begin the practice of true, spiritual journaling…

Do This:

1. Have a place to keep your private, written thoughts.

Ever since Adam and Eve, we've been ducking for cover, haven't we? But absolute honesty before God and ourselves is the key to making this practice work for you. And if you're nervous about someone reading your uncensored thoughts—and we all are—you won't be completely candid. So, have a place where you can keep your journals under lock and key.

2. Set aside a regular time and a quiet place.

As with the practice of contemplative quiet, the more often you do this and the less you're distracted, the more benefit you'll gain.

3. Let your thoughts begin to flow.

You don't need to set out with a topic in mind. This is not college theme writing. As you sit quietly, pick a topic out of the air—any one of those little thought-bubbles that pop spontaneously out of your head.

Today, it may be a tiny little worry about one of your children, or a relationship…. Follow it down to its source in your spirit by asking: What am I afraid is going wrong? What have I been doing to try to fix things? Where do I feel powerless—and what can I do about this sense of powerlessness? What part do I trust to God—and what's my part?

Tomorrow, your focus may be on a problem in your community, or on the job. Follow the sense of conflict or injustice or challenge down to its source in your spirit by asking: What issues are at odds here? What are my values telling me? What are my values telling me to *do* about what's wrong? If I can't correct the problem by myself—who else can I join with? And what can we realistically accomplish?

Let the thoughts…flow.

4. Don't let censoring voices shut you down.

Sometimes voices in our heads tell us we shouldn't be thinking or feeling what we really are feeling. Maybe we've internalized the voice of Mother or Dad or some other stern, cautionary voice. If we give in to this voice that labels our own thoughts and soul-content as "forbidden" we will not get down to many of the deep-level stresses that are conflicting our spirits...and that's bad news for our well-being.

So...on days when you get down to those highly personal issues—say, manipulations you know you're using in relation-ships...or matters of sexuality...or honest misgivings about a person you know...or the truth about your feelings toward someone you feel you should love (but you don't)...*have courage.*

Open your spirit to God. God *already* knows what you've been thinking and feeling, and He has just been waiting for you to come around and admit it. *Only* when we reach this ground-zero in our spirit can we begin to build our life on a stable foundation of hon-esty and intent.

5. Every month, review your journal.

Hindsight usually leads to insight. As we look back over a month's worth of deep-level honesty, we begin to connect the dots. We see themes—reminding us of what we really value, warning us not to ignore intuitions about certain people and sit-uations, focusing us in on what the real core issues are in impor-tant relationships. We start to learn what to say *no* to...and what to say *yes* to.

In short, we connect with our own spirit again. We live out of a sense of values and beliefs...not stretched thin and pulled apart by life's demands.

The benefits to someone struggling with PMS are substantial: You've added another practice that's creating a state of inner calm—reducing the stress in your body, *and* you've fortified your mind against those emotional crashes that come when PMS symp-toms amplify the message that your life is going nowhere, and you're not growing. Now you *are* growing...and your life *is* going somewhere.

Strategy #4: Confession—Taking the Weight Off

An old and very accurate saying says, "Confession is good for the soul."

Sometimes we can confront ourselves all we want and even point directly at the exact things we're doing wrong that mess up our lives. We can see it—sort of—but then we don't *do* anything to change what we see.

Welcome to more deep-level conflict in our spirit. Like other deep-level conflicts, the sense that you've grievously hurt or let down other people is most likely to surface on days when PMS has jarred every nerve. Unfortunately, you're not in a place to really *do* much to resolve the problem, and you're merely victimized by the turmoil.

The spiritual practice of confession is a great way to release and resolve stress in our spirit. Even if this practice is not part of your tradition, you can benefit from it.

Do This:

Build a confessional relationship with someone who will guard your deepest secrets and count every journey into your open spirit as sacred.

Some women rely on counselors for this, others seek help from the clergy. Make it clear you are mainly looking for someone who can...

- listen to your honest confession without pronouncing judgment

- help you see clearly what you're doing wrong

- not let you get away with excusing your behavior ("I really *had* to lie because...") or with blaming the other person ("She has everything, that's why I gossip about her...." "My husband makes me so frustrated, I *had* to cheat....")

- help you peg your *real* motives ("I'm too gutless to ask for what I want because I'm afraid I won't get it exactly my way so I manipulate by…")

- help you to recognize more honest, forthright, and spiritually mature ways to live so that you're not harming other people by your actions…and harming your spirit by these subterfuges.

A confessional relationship is not the same as "a good talk" with a close friend. A confessional relationship begins and ends with committing all that's spoken about to God. All that passes is held in complete confidence.

Most important, God's presence is invoked by prayer. And the "confessor" will also close your time by offering the forgiveness of God…and prayer that grace will help you grow and change.

Those who have never experienced a confessional relationship will be amazed at the overall benefits to spirit, mind, *and* body this kind of relationship offers.

Strategy #5: Sacred Reading

Lectio divina—sacred reading—is another wonderful, old, spiritual practice that offers us overall health benefits. Wise, insightful, inspiring words are like remedies for what ails us in spirit.

In the third century, "mothers" of the church noted that sacred reading empowers the inner person in a way that "sends all manner of evils fleeing"—including many physical ailments. Hildegard of Bingen, an abbess and herbalist of the eleventh century, also prescribed sacred reading for those who came to her seeking treatment for their ailments. And actually, the belief that sacred reading has healing virtues has been around since much earlier times.

Life's challenges are constantly wearing on us. Everyday demands grind us down. Trouble and evil in the world leave us with fear and anxiety. Circumstances catch us by surprise, and we lack the wisdom and experience to handle difficulties and complexities. We feel bombarded and overwhelmed. Add to this the constant inner challenges you face when your monthly cycle is torturing you, making you feel like a mental, spiritual, and physical disaster.

Sacred reading soothes and fortifies the inner being. Here are two types of reading you'll want to try as you create your own "apothecary of the spirit":

Scriptures

Many biblical writings are refreshing for their honesty and authenticity about human experience...for their ability to give voice to our deepest feelings, thoughts, questions, and conflicts. Some are challenging, and some have a tonic effect. Some just have the rare ability to lift the spirit.

Many passages throughout the Bible will speak to you. But for a sacred reading experience that's spirit lifting and healing, begin or end your day with selections like the following:

Psalm 5...when you need assurances that God is close and listening to you.

Psalm 11...speaks of our spirit's "refuge" and place of security in God.

Psalm 23...when you feel anxious.

Psalm 32...assures us we *are* forgiven...and that God is patient in growing us up.

Psalm 62...when your soul is agitated and needs focus and quiet rest.

Psalm 84...when inner turmoil has robbed you of a sense that life is good.

Psalm 102...when you are in deep distress.

Psalm 124...when financial and other woes of life are burdening you.

Psalm 139...when you need assurance that God loves *you*.

Luke 1:46-55..."Mary's Song"...for a reminder that your life is important and purposeful.

Romans 8...when many problems, challenges, and obstacles are stacked against you.

1 Corinthians 13...to remind you that God's love for you is like no other love.

Inspirational Writings

Besides the scriptures, many people of faith have written profoundly wise and inspiring works that are spiritually "restorative" like a good tonic

Here are a few great writings by valiant women of faith whose words will have a tonic effect on your spirit:

Revelations of Divine Love (or *Showings*) by Julian of Norwich

The Interior Castle by Teresa of Avilla

The Christian's Secret of a Happy Life by Hannah Whitall Smith

Candles in the Dark by Amy Carmichael

Pilgrim at Tinker Creek by Annie Dillard

The Cloister Walk by Kathleen Norris

A Final Word About Your Spirit

One of the greatest spiritual stresses some women suffer is the sense that their life has little or no purpose. When PMS symptoms hit, this aimless feeling can open up like a chasm...and life can feel terrifyingly empty and meaningless.

The truth is, every woman's life has a purpose—a *meaningful* purpose that brings great fulfillment when it's found. For some the purpose can be as simple as creating a home for a family. Some women feel destined to use their gifts in the service of others. Still others sense a calling to places of creativity, business, leadership, and example. In each case, the exact nature of the purpose isn't as important as the woman's discovery and pursuit of her destiny.

A woman who acknowledges and cultivates her spiritual nature will have a head start in the management of any bodily distraction, including PMS. As you employ the spiritual strategies in this chapter, don't be surprised if new desires and even opportunities to pursue your personal purpose in life appear.

No matter what your calling as a woman...finding the path that leads to fulfillment can gain you an advantage in controlling the distraction of PMS.

4

The PMS Diet

C hoosing an appropriate diet is one of the most important (and neglected) strategies you can use for controlling PMS. Knowing which foods to avoid and which ones to emphasize will help you go a long way toward relieving those awful symptoms. Eating the right foods can help you...

→ balance wildly fluctuating hormones and restore calm and control

→ eliminate toxins that cause stomach and digestive distress and even trigger headaches

→ introduce "food medicines" that relieve cramps and inhibit potential tumor growth

→ boost your body and restore energy

Begin with a Great Diet

In this chapter, the emphasis is on eating a well-balanced diet. A good diet is one that includes the right percentages of the best proteins, complex carbohydrates, and fats. You can't eat a poor or unbalanced diet and expect to throw a few health foods down the gullet to get the results you want.

So although the foods highlighted here are part of the diet for women who want to successfully control PMS, take note of the overall dietary instructions throughout. These recommendations are the foundation on which you need to build to see the maximum health benefit from the specific foods mentioned.

Strategy #1: Use Complex Carbs as "Food Medicine"

Complex carbohydrates—which we get from fruits, grains, and vegetables—are extremely important in the diet of a woman with PMS. Complex carbs contain thousands of phytochemicals essential for optimum health...or for correcting a health condition. These natural compounds are so vital to our well-being they're often considered to be natural medicine in food form.

Many natural healthcare practitioners, in fact, highly recommend that women with PMS eat a vegetarian diet...but because that's probably not practical or desirable for most women, let's talk about a more realistic approach.

You can experience great health benefits if you balance your diet so that about **40 percent of your calories come from the complex carbs** in fruits, grains, and vegetables. Plan to eat far fewer simple carbs like pastas and breads.

In each of these categories though, some food items are much better choices than others. The foods recommended here are known to be rich in phytochemicals that contribute to better health, which is why they're highly recommended to you if you're dealing with PMS symptoms.

Fruits

The variety and amount of fruit available to us assures many healthy choices at our fingertips. Fruit makes the best snack. Unfortunately, most of us reach for the chips, nuts, cookies, baked goods, candy bars....

Here's why you need to eat more fruit.

- Given the fact that most snack items are in the "problem food" category for women with PMS (see pages 53-54), fruits are, at the very least, important as snack foods. But that's not the end of it, not by far.

- Fruits are high in dietary fiber, important for digestion.

- Fruits are storehouses of cancer-fighting phytochemicals that work overtime to counter the carcinogenic dangers of too much estrogen.

- Eating more fruit promotes health in the urinary tract.

- Fruits are loaded with essential vitamins and minerals.

Not all fruits are equally beneficial for you if you're specifically eating to control PMS. **Apples** and **pears** are more ph-basic, and if yeast infections are a common problem you want to keep your system slightly more acidic…so go light on these two.

The fruits listed below are high in carotenoids, beta-carotene, bioflavanoids, and anthocyanins. This places them among your best complex-carb choices for a PMS-controlling diet.

apricots	mangoes
blueberries	papayas
citrus	peaches
grapes	strawberries

These fruits have an added benefit for those who are concerned about cancer: They are high in antioxidants, which help cleanse the blood of free radicals known to trigger cancer.

Grains

Actually, we need to back up a step before recommending any grains.

For years, the U.S. Food and Drug Administration has recommended that we eat several hefty servings of grains and cereals each day. At the same time, other branches of the government issued warnings that as a population we are getting…well…*hefty*.

Recently, doctors and nutritionists have pointed out many serious health problems caused by the government's dietary recommendations. For one thing we shouldn't be eating nearly as much grain as recommended, especially in the more refined forms like flour. In a nutshell, if you eat too many grain-based foods along with other simple carbohydrates, you trigger reactions in the body that result in continual weight gain. As one leading doctor, an expert in diet and nutrition, put it, "What do you think they feed cattle to fatten them just before slaughter?" Grain, of course.

So although certain grains are good dietary sources of nutrients that ease PMS symptoms, it's recommended you use them lightly. Weight gain is not good for overall health. And if you're struggling with PMS, you don't need the added stress of having your self-image and self-esteem challenged by weight gain.

Nonetheless, some whole grains—in modest amounts—can become an important part of your diet. Here are the ones that will offer you the most benefit.

- **Barley** is as high in protein as meats. It's versatile and can be eaten as a cooked cereal, mixed into soup, or baked into whole-grain breads. The phytochemicals in barley help regulate hormone production and can prevent tumor growth.

- **Brown Rice.** Nutritionally, whole-grain brown rice bears little resemblance to its cousin—sticky white rice. Brown rice is high in the antioxidant minerals selenium and zinc and in the bone-building minerals phosphorous and magnesium. It's also a great source of energy because it's rich in B vitamins, and it falls in the middle of the glycemic index so it won't make your blood-sugar levels spike and drop. High in fiber, it also cleanses the colon. Some consider it a near-perfect complex carb.

- **Quinoa.** From the Andes, quinoa (*keen*-wah) has the highest protein of any grain at 16 percent. It's a complete protein with an amino acid profile much like milk. It's also high in iron for blood-building, in the B vitamins, and in Vitamin E. Quinoa is very easy to digest, making its energy quickly available to your body. Black quinoa has an even richer, nuttier flavor than white. Either one can be substituted for rice, millet, or couscous in cooking.

- **Soy.** Normally, soy flour would be a good substitute for white flour in baking but soy promotes estrogen production, which can make it a problem for many women. (See Proteins, pg. 59.)

- **Spelt** is a good substitute for white flour in baking. In breads it has a flavor something like sourdough without being a potential headache trigger like sourdough.

Vegetables

Veggies are an excellent source of complex carbohydrates as well as many important vitamins, minerals, and other phytochemicals. Here are some of the best choices:

- *The Dark Green Leafy Ones.* The dark green vegetables contain large amounts of beta-carotene, which has a tonic effect on your immune system and contributes to gynecological health. They also contain high amounts of Vitamin K and other vitamins, plus magnesium, zinc, and numerous other minerals.

  The vegetables in this category also contain indoles, which help produce enzymes that neutralize the harmful effects of too much estrogen—making them important if you want to increase your resistance to breast, ovarian, and other types of cancer. The top veggies to choose in this category are

broccoli	sea kelp
brussels sprouts	spinach
cabbage	turnip greens
kale	

- *The Red Ones.* Red vegetables also contain beta-carotene as well as the carotenoid known as lutein, another important immune booster and cancer fighter. (And it promotes good vision.) Best choices are

beets	tomatoes
red peppers	

- *The Yellow and Orange Ones.* This category contains the important carotenoids and beta-carotenes in spades, along with other immune-boosting and cancer-preventing phytochemicals. Choose:

carrots	yellow peppers
squash	yams

- *The Little Round Ones (Beans and Legumes).* If bloating and digestive troubles are a real problem, you'll want to minimize these in your diet. Otherwise...

  Beans are high in water-soluble fiber, good for bonding with waste products and moving them quickly out of the body. There is, of course, that one small problem—but it can be handled by mixing mint (dried or fresh) with your bean dishes or using Bean-O™. Beans and legumes are high in protein, low in fat, and the phytochemicals in them have tonic effects on internal organs such as the stomach, spleen, liver, and pancreas. They also offer cancer-resisting benefits. If you can eat beans, your best choices are

  adzuki beans (hokaidos)

  chickpeas (garbanzos)

  dark red kidney beans

  wax beans

- *The Starchy Ones.* Starchy vegetables like potatoes and corn should be very low on your list. They slow down digestion and trigger insulin production, which contributes to weight gain and makes you more susceptible to diabetes. Limiting or doing without them will not harm you.

℞
PROBLEM FOODS

∼

Certain foods cause real problems for women with PMS. Some on this list may be obvious—others may surprise you.

Alcohol. This wreaks havoc with your brain chemistry, hormone production, blood pressure, digestion, urinary tract…need we keep going? Moderation is not even the key. If you want to drink alcohol—*a few sips* is the key. During the worst part of your cycle, though, alcohol should be totally off-limits.

Butter. There are much healthier dietary choices for the healthy fats you need in your diet. Also butter is rich and contributes to sluggish digestion and nausea.

Caffeine. Obvious, right? If you're fighting the mood roller coaster, a jolt of caffeine—whether from coffee or cola drinks—is a bad choice. If your excuse is that you need an energy boost…can't support you there either. Eating smaller, better meals more often and snacking on fruits and other energy-boosting foods is the healthy way to keep energy balanced throughout the day.

Chocolate. (Send all complaints to: P.O. Box Z, South Pole.) Sorry, but the caffeine, sugar, and fat in chocolate can wreak havoc with a woman's hormonal levels, affecting her moods and energy levels.

Dairy. Dairy products can cause digestive problems during the most difficult parts of your cycle. In addition, certain cheeses—the aged ones like Blue and Roquefort—can trigger headaches and migraines.

Fried Foods. These are bad for the digestion, and they introduce too many acids into your system, which puts an extra demand on hormone production—which is already a problem.

MSG (monosodium glutamate). MSG has been linked to vascular headaches and migraines. With hormones affecting your cardiovascular system, be very careful about this additive, which is hidden in many processed foods, sometimes as a "natural flavoring."

Salt (in excess). A little salt is usually fine. But if high blood pressure and/or water retention are problems, you may need to avoid salt altogether. Really good salt substitutes exist. Use them instead.

Refined Sugar. In women with PMS and other menstrual or gynecological problems, sugar is perhaps the most common trigger of yeast infections. If sugar substitutes are a problem for you, try unrefined sugars.

White Flour. The gluten in white flour is a problem for many people to begin with. Add to that the fact that foods made with white flour trigger hormonal responses that cause weight gain, digestive sluggishness, and other physical problems, and white flour becomes a poor dietary choice.

If any of these foods are on your personal "I can't live without this" list…then at least try to avoid them as much as possible during the ten days before your period.

Strategy #2: Use Fats for Flavor...Sparingly

Thanks to the multi-billion-dollar dieting and beauty industries, too many women have a terrible relationship with their bodies and their physical appearance. As a result, many women experience emotional discomfort ranging from mild to extreme when the topic of the fats in our foods come up. On one extreme are women who drive themselves insane keeping fat out of their diet. On the other extreme are those who have gotten tired of fighting it and mostly ignore their fat intake.

It's time for a bit of wise balance.

Fat is an essential part of a healthy diet. Even if you're trying to lose weight, you actually need some fat in your diet in order to build the hormones that target and burn the fat stored on your body. (A zero-fat diet is *not* a healthy diet.) We also need some fat in our diet to make fat-soluble vitamins—like A, D, E, and K—do their important work. Fat is also needed to trigger the production of various hormones.

The simple keys to using dietary fats wisely—for overall well-being and in controlling PMS—are these:

1. Eat the right kinds of fat.

2. Eat fat in small amounts.

As a rule of thumb, about *30 percent* **of your calories should come from fats.** That sounds like a lot, but because fats are so calorie-rich, the amount of fat you put into your diet is actually going to look very small compared to the amount of complex carbohydrates and proteins you eat.

For example, you need to eat a good-sized serving of salad to get the right amount of complex carbs you need...while you need only a little more than a tablespoon of most salad dressings to reach your maximum fat need for the same meal.

Women who fight PMS often have too much fat in their diets. Remember, fats—especially the wrong kind—trigger an overproduction of hormones and also throw off your digestion. What fats are least beneficial, then? They are...

➔ **animal fat—especially from red meats**

➔ **monounsaturated fats—found in cottonseed, soy, and tropical cooking oils**

If these are the fats to be avoided, then what are the better choices? They include...

Butters

If you're serious about switching products, you can substitute certain oils for butter in your recipes. If you absolutely crave the taste of butter, or you can't substitute in a recipe, check your grocery store's dairy case for the new **butter and olive oil** blends. They're much better for you, and you won't even notice the mild olive flavor in your cooking.

Although you'll find good old-fashioned butter on the list of foods that can be a problem for PMS sufferers, not *all* butters are a problem. It's time to branch out. Besides the substitute mentioned above, your better choices are

almond butter   **natural peanut butter**

cashew butter

And your very best choices are seed butters like

> **sesame butter**
>
> **sunflower butter**

Though you may find **soy butter** for sale in health food stores, it is actually of very poor nutritional value. Skip it.

Nuts

Okay, so you already know that nuts are loaded with fat.

That doesn't mean you can't have them ground as a garnish, say, on top of a salad. Or eat a few along with fish or poultry and vegetables to add the small amount of fat needed to balance out a great, healthy meal.

The best choices are:

> **almonds**   **cashews**
>
> **brazil nuts**   **macadamias**

Chopping or slivering three or four nuts *max* and sprinkling them on salad, fish, or poultry gives you a little bit of sweet flavor and all the fat you need at that meal.

Culinary Oils

The oils you want are the ones high in omega-3 fatty acids (EFAs). They don't become toxic in your system as do other oils used widely in our foods. Best choices?

- **Olive Oil.** This one is the most widely used, especially the "extra virgin" variety. It's low in saturated fats and high in EFAs. It also supports liver and gallbladder function.

- **Sesame Oil** is another top choice. Readily available in grocery stores, it's high in the antioxidant Vitamin E and has as much iron as liver. It's also high in two important amino acids, making it a source of vegetable protein, too.

Oils to eliminate? Though **canola oil** is highly touted as a healthy choice because it doesn't increase cholesterol, it can become mildly toxic in your body due to its high refinement and low EFA content. **Corn oil** is nutritionally valueless. And tropicals, such as **coconut oil** and **palm oil** are high in saturated fats, which will send your cholesterol soaring.

If you have cancer or are concerned about it because of family history or a past bout with it, healthcare experts recommend that you keep your fat intake lower than normal…at just *10* to *15 percent* of your total diet.

FRIENDLY BACTERIA

~

Your intestinal and urinary tracts and your vagina are inhabited by strains of bacteria that are beneficial to your body. They help with digestion, produce Vitamin B, kill disease-causing bacteria, and boost immunity.

Many factors, however, can wipe out these microscopic allies: antibiotics and other strong medicines such as cortisone, birth control pills and lubricants, too much candy or sugar in your diet, and plain old stress. (You don't have any stress in your life, do you?) When the good bacteria is wiped out, other harmful bacteria can take over. Enter *candida albicans*, and you have an unpleasant yeast infection.

To restore or maintain the friendly bacteria naturally…

1. *Eat a diet rich in fruits, vegetables, whole grains, and in foods with bacteria cultures like activated yogurt.*

2. *Take probiotics, available in supplement form in health food stores.*

If you go with a supplement…buy the *soft capsules* because the process that produces probiotics in *hard caplets* can reduce potency. And buy the bottle with the most recent date and the greatest potency.

Strategy #3: Maintain Balance...with Proteins

Eating the right kinds of proteins can help you make big gains on PMS.

In general, certain types of proteins promote overall health, while others stress the digestive system, tax your hormonal output, and circulate acid and toxins throughout the body.

To eat a well-balanced diet, about *30 percent* **of your calories should come from proteins.** What are poor protein choices, and which are better options?

Red Meats

This is a protein source you should limit if you're serious about wanting relief from PMS symptoms.

In fact, we're all far better off treating red meats as a garnish rather than a main course. If you love an occasional London broil or prime rib—okay. But red meat is actually a poor choice for a healthy diet, especially for women.

The protein in red meat contains higher amounts of the omega-6 fatty acids—the kind we know as "bad cholesterol," which promotes tumor growth and heart disease.

If that's not enough, red meat is hard to digest. This puts a big strain on the body's hormone production. Welcome greater mood swings. And because so much digestive acid is required to process red meat, your body may actually begin to "mine" from your bones the raw ingredients needed to make extra acid. Welcome osteoporosis.

Other protein sources are much healthier choices.

Vegetable Protein

Several plants top the dietary lists as sources of proteins.

Women with PMS should go back and look at the **grains** mentioned, and at the **beans and legumes** as well. Lots of good plant protein is mixed in with those complex carbs.

Soy foods are an excellent source of plant-based protein. Because soy is so widely used in health foods, it needs special mention in the context of controlling PMS. There are plus and minus sides to soy.

+ Soy is rich in protein and easy to digest, making its nutrition and energy readily available. It's also a great source of gen-estein, a substance that blocks the flow of blood to tumors. It's widely used and available in many forms: **soy milk, tofu, soy burgers, soy mayonnaise, soy sausage, soy bacon, soy yogurt.** It's also an ingredient in **miso**, an oriental paste used in making delicious soups and sauces.

− Soy has a mild, estriol-like effect in your body, which means it promotes the production of estrogen. (If you're going to use it in cooking for the family, do not tell your husband or sons this.) If over-production of estrogen is a problem, then you will want to be careful in how much soy you add to your diet.

All factors considered, though, getting your protein from soy, among other plant sources, is a far better alternative than getting it from red meat…and it still ranks ahead of the next best protein sources.

Fish

In cultures where fish is the main source of dietary protein, studies have shown that people are healthier by far. Not only is there a much lower incidence of cancer and heart disease, women also experience fewer gynecological and menstrual problems.

Fish are high in the omega-3 fatty acids and other nutrients such as vitamins B_6, B_{12}, and folic acid, which help prevent tumors from forming.

Here is a list of recommended fish and other seafoods with those containing the most EFAs at the top:

><> **anchovies, herring, mackerel, salmon**

><> **albacore tuna, sablefish, sardines**

><> **bluefin tuna, trout**

><> **halibut, swordfish**

><> **freshwater bass, oysters**

><> sea bass

><> pollock, shrimp

><> catfish, crabs

><> clams, cod, flounder, scallops

Poultry

Although we've been trained to think of poultry—"the white meat"—as a healthier choice than red meats, that can be untrue, depending on which brands you buy. *Read those labels.* Some poultry is actually loaded with unhealthy fat.

Here's what to look for:

- **Chicken.** Look for free-range chicken, especially the kind raised on grain containing DHA, which gives the meat a better balance of fatty acids. If chickens are fed with DHA, you'll find the information on the label.

- **Turkey.** Again, choose the free-range brands, raised on grain containing DHA. Besides being a good protein source, turkey is high in tryptophan, a naturally-occurring amino acid needed for the brain's production of neurotransmitter chemicals. Turkey is not exactly a mood-boosting food by itself, but it does support good mental health as well as physical health.

- **Eggs.** The eggs from free-range chickens are your best choice. If they come from chickens raised on the special feed just mentioned they will contain that important balance of the EFAs.

Strategy #4: A Nice Cup of Tea...and Other Good Drinks

The fact is, we should all be drinking more water and natural drinks. It's also a great idea to eliminate carbonated soft drinks and highly processed fruit juices as much as possible, because they're loaded with empty calories and unhealthy corn sweeteners.

When you're experiencing PMS symptoms, your body is naturally under stress, and you're likely to be mildly to moderately dehydrated...not to mention feeling exhausted. Aside from good old water, your best choices are...

- **Almond Milk.** This is a flavorful alternative to cows' milk, and it contains a cyanide-like natural substance that isn't toxic to anything in your body but pre-cancerous cells and tumors.

- **Fruit Shakes.** Great for a mid-morning or mid-afternoon lift, fruit shakes boost your energy and flood your body with antioxidants, enzymes, minerals, phytochemicals, and vitamins. They can be made ahead, carried along in a thermos and re-shaken before drinking. Making these shakes with almond milk increases the health benefits.

- **Teas.** At last...the "nice cup of tea" part. Teas have been important in natural medicines for many centuries. They also offer the comfort of a warm cup or mug to cradle in your hands and a bit of nurturing warmth in the tummy, too.

  Green tea is by far the favorite infusion of health-conscious people everywhere. Green tea is rich in antioxidants and other substances that work at the cellular level to inhibit tumor growth, and it is a whole-body tonic as well. Green tea is sold pre-bagged and in loose form, ready to be spooned into your tea ball.

Here are two recipes for other infusions—both made of ingredients that relieve PMS symptoms:

Recipe 1: Delicious Raspberry-Clover—a "Mood" Tea

> 1 ounce red raspberry leaves
> 1 ounce red clover
> 1 ounce chamomile (optional)
> 1 quart water

The leaves of the red raspberry help ease the effects of hormonal fluctuations throughout your cycle, and they're high in Vitamin C and calcium. Red clover has nerve-soothing properties and is high in calcium and magnesium. Add chamomile, and this makes a wonderful bedtime drink.

Recipe 2: Ginger-Mint Tea—to Soothe the Body

1 ounce grated fresh ginger root
1 ounce peppermint
1 quart water

For centuries ginger root has been used as a folk medicine for upset stomachs and unsettled digestion...and for women who suffer from cramping during their cycle. The mint adds a cool refreshment to the zing of the ginger.

5

Nature's Apothecary

Some of the supplemental remedies discussed in this chapter are known to react with particular medications. Others may have adverse effects on certain health conditions—such as pregnancy, mood or anxiety disorders, or physical disorders such as diabetes or high blood pressure.

As each supplement is discussed, some but not all contraindications are mentioned. You should check with a healthcare professional and/or your pharmacist to ask which supplements are safe and right for you.

Many women are turning to natural supplements—vitamins, herbs, hormones, minerals, and other products—to ease the symptoms of PMS.

Perhaps you've picked up on the controversies surrounding the use of natural supplements. Let's take a moment to consider this controversy.

Natural Remedies...the Questions

TV news magazines run regular features on vitamins, herbs, minerals, or other natural substances that are misused or overused. On one side of the issue will be an official from a government bureau that regulates healthcare matters who will denounce the use of natural supplements as "dangerous" at worst and "a waste of your money" at best. He'll lobby for more regulation of natural supplements by the government. On the other side of the issue will be perhaps a naturopathic doctor...and usually someone claiming to be cured by natural supplements who will insist that natural reme-dies restored her health. Sometimes the stories of recovery are dra-matic and convincing.

Natural remedies are continually being subjected to ongoing scientific tests—even as you read this. Some are proving to be effec-tive in managing or curing the conditions they claim to help. Others are proving to be weak or not effective at all.

Interestingly, members of the traditional medical community and responsible practitioners of natural medicine share some of the same concerns when it comes to the use of natural supplements.

- Some manufacturers do not provide adequate quality control testing on their products. This means that depending on the company whose supplement you're using, the therapeutic dose can vary widely from batch to batch—even capsule to capsule in the same batch or bottle. Some doses may actually contain *none* of the active ingredient you're counting on to relieve your symptoms.

- When many of us read "natural" on a label, we assume that means a product is entirely safe. In fact, some natural sup-plements, most notably herbs, are known to react with med-ications and even with other herbs. Often, this specific information is *not* printed on the labels or product inserts of natural products.

- Some users of natural remedies show a careless disregard in their use of products. Some "mix and match" natural reme-dies until it's difficult, if not impossible, to tell which product is being effective. Others are impatient and don't try a product long enough to allow its active ingredients to reach a therapeutic level in their bodies.

- Finally—and this a main complaint of traditional health-care practitioners—much of the evidence that natural reme-dies work is "anecdotal." Not enough scientific studies have been completed at this point (keep in mind they take many years) for the official medical community to agree that claims made about a natural remedy are valid.

Most natural healthcare practitioners part company with the medical community on this last point. Many, many thousands of people are reporting that they've been cured or their symptoms have been eased by using natural supplements. That fact, supporters and users say, is enough evidence to go on. Why should people wait around, suffering for years, waiting for studies to be completed when help is at hand?

Wise Answers

Natural remedies *are* effective. No one questions the fact that vitamins, herbs, natural hormones, or minerals *do* affect body chemistry and alter body processes—sometimes powerfully.

Because people are turning to these alternatives, we need answers to the bigger question: How can we be wise in our use of them so that we don't cause harm to ourselves…*and* so that we do get the maximum benefit from the ones that are effective?

Here are some guidelines for the wise use of natural supplements:

1. Learn if there are any side-effects or if any health conditions you have are affected by the use of this supplement.

2. Unless it's recommended that you take supplements in combination (for example calcium, potassium, and magnesium), take only one supplement at a time to treat a given symptom.

3. Drink water throughout the day when taking supplements—not just the glass you drink at the time you take them. Your liver and kidneys will need extra water to function well when you're taking supplements.

4. Give it time. It can take two or three weeks for the active ingredient in a supplement to reach its therapeutic level in your body. If after a month a product does not seem to be helping, consider switching to another.

5. Be observant of your body. When you first start taking a supplement, stay alert to possible side effects. Some can happen quickly…as in the case of the well-known B_6 (niacin) flush, which is harmless. If you experience unpleasant side effects,

discontinue use immediately and flush your system with water.

6. Write down what you are taking. In the event of a medical emergency, or even a routine doctor's visit, medical personnel must know everything you've been taking in order to treat you properly and avoid dangerous or unpleasant drug-supplement reactions.

By following these simple steps, you can avoid difficulties and get the maximum benefits out of the natural supplements you use to combat PMS.

The Natural Remedies

The Herb Shelf

Herbs played an important role in "folk medicine" for many centuries, long before the advent of our powerful and fast-acting synthetic pharmaceuticals in the twentieth century. These modern pharmaceuticals, however, are more likely to have side effects and may even cause long-term damage. Of course, sometimes you will need these prescription drugs, and when you use them you're wise to ask about their side effects…and also ask what you can do to counter them.

In the past three decades, the rising interest in "natural medicine" has turned a spotlight back on the use of herbs. Actually, this return to using herbal medicines applies only to the United States. In most of the rest of the world, interest in and use of herbs was never abandoned.

Numerous studies have now been completed, and more are under way, proving the effectiveness of many herbal remedies. Some have been found to work just as effectively as prescription drugs, though their active ingredients are less concentrated, and thus they take longer to reach a therapeutic level in your system. Testing has also allowed us, at this point, to dismiss fraudulent or over-inflated claims about some herbs—also to identify, among those that do work, which ones interact unfavorably with certain prescription drugs.

Fortunately, a number of herbs offer great relief to the woman suffering from PMS. A few are overall tonics. Some can help you even out your whole menstrual cycle and can be taken all the time (though a few need to be avoided during your period). Others will help you find great relief from specific symptoms such as cramping, headaches, or mood swings.

The herbs listed following are tried-and-true remedies, many of them used by women for centuries.

- *Black Cohosh.* Though this herb is often used in higher doses to treat post-menopausal women, it has benefits when taken in normal doses by menstruating women as well. It has an estriol-like effect, simulating the effects of estrogen (in milder form) on the body.

  You will need to work with this herb carefully, and also with any other herbs that produce an estriol-like effect. If your estrogen levels drop to abnormally low levels during part of your cycle, you should use them only during that time. Obviously, if your estrogen levels are always on the high side, you should not use this herb or others that stimulate its further production.

  Some readers will want to keep Black Cohosh in mind and come back to it later, after menopause, to prevent vaginal atrophy.

  Black Cohosh is available in an extract form and in dried form in capsules.

- *Chamomile and Chamomile Oil.* Chamomile contains compounds that relieve cramps and promote healthy menstrual flow. This herb is often drunk as a tea—usually at nap-time or at night because it promotes sleep. The dried herb can also be taken in capsule form.

  In addition, some herbalists recommend rubbing essential chamomile oil directly into the abdomen for cramp relief. *Do not take chamomile oil internally.*

- *Cramp Bark*...is also known by a more pleasant name— **Black Haw**. Lydia Pinkham's Vegetable Compound, one of the most popular women's elixirs of the nineteenth and early twentieth centuries, contained this legendary herb, whose benefits as a muscle relaxant were discovered by early Native Americans. Besides being an effective cramp-reliever (hence, the name), its overall anti-stress and anti-anxiety properties are well-known.

Cramp Bark is considered most effective in extract form, though it is also available in dried form in capsules.

- *Dong Quai* (*a.k.a.* **Female Ginseng**). This amazing herb is a phyto-estrogen—that is, estrogen from a plant source. It has been widely used in the east for centuries to regulate a woman's cycle. Because of its hormone-stabilizing effects, Dong Quai helps to keep your energy balanced, which means you may no longer experience those sudden dips and that awful, wiped-out feeling.

Although herbalists highly recommend the use of this herb for most of your cycle, they recommend that you *not* use Dong Quai once your actual period begins. That's because it tends to stimulate more-than-normal blood flow. Resume use again once your period has stopped.

Herbalists most often recommend taking Dong Quai in extract form.

- *Feverfew*...comes from the aster family, and from ancient to more recent times has been known as something of a wonder drug, curing both headaches and "melancholy." Its main active ingredient is parthenolide and is most effective when taken on a regular basis rather than the moment a headache or darker mood strikes.

Feverfew is available in capsules and in raw leaf form.

Note: *This herb should not be used during pregnancy as it is known to bring on menses. It can also affect blood-clotting, so you should not use it before or after surgery or if you are taking a blood-thinning medication such as Coumadin or Warfarin.*

- *Ginger Root.* Okay, so maybe you're carrying gingersnaps in your car in case you or the kids get queasy in the stomach. Ginger root has more potent medicinal uses due to the healing properties of its most active ingredient, gingerol. In fact, Ginger root has been used for centuries to help women ward off even the most painful cramps of menstruation.

  You will want to use the fresh root, shredded into a tea ball, to make a flavorful, pain-relieving tea.

- *Kava.* Though the western healthcare community has been slow to acknowledge the effectiveness of many herbal remedies, this one has quickly gained a reasonably good reputation. The fast, anxiety-reducing benefits of Kava have been compared to benzodiazapene drugs like Ativan, Valium, and Xanax—but, of course, it's natural.

  Additionally, it relieves even strong muscle cramps and is a powerful mood elevator.

  Note: Kava should never be taken if you are using alcohol or prescription sedatives. It will increase the effectiveness of other sleep- and relaxation-inducing supplements. It should also not be taken by women with Parkinson's Disease.

  Caution: Recent reports from Europe are suggesting a possible link between Kava use and liver damage. Check with a healthcare professional before using Kava.

- *Licorice Root.* Licorice root stimulates the adrenal glands, thus helping to regulate hormone production throughout your cycle.

  This herb stimulates your whole system, causing your body to expel excess mucous. For that reason it's often used to relieve colds, allergies, and sinus infections. It also helps promote quicker, more thorough shedding of the uterine lining during your period.

  Licorice root is available in capsules and in extract. It makes a wonderful, flavorful tea—which is always a comfort when you're feeling generally lousy, isn't it?

- *Meadowsweet.* The word *aspirin* comes from *spirea*, which is an alternate name for meadowsweet. What's the connection? Meadowsweet contains salicylin, which the body converts to salicylic acid, the active ingredient in aspirin.

  Meadowsweet offers a much gentler, safer alternative to aspirin. Yes, it may take a few minutes longer for the herb to counter your headache, but it's also less destructive to your stomach lining. Additionally, meadowsweet can help relieve lower back pain sometimes associated with PMS.

  Meadowsweet tea is a common way to ingest this herb, which is available in dried form and in extract.

- *Raspberry Leaf.* If your menstrual cramping is not sporadic, but extends through most of your period, raspberry leaf might be the right herb for you. Its active agents relax the muscles that cause cramping. Raspberry leaf is rich in calcium, magnesium, and iron, which contribute to the health of your reproductive organs.

  Raspberry leaf is available as an extract or in dried form and can be taken as a tea.

- *Rhodiola.* This is one of the most effective herbs to take if you find yourself overwhelmed, under unbearable stress, and need immediate relief. If you are given to panic attacks you may wish to try rhodiola at the first signs of attack, in place of intervention drugs like Lorazepam.

  Rhodiola is an adaptogen, which means it acts as a whole-body tonic to increase your resistance to physical, emotional, and chemical stressors. Its other great benefit is that it increases the production of serotonin in your brain, causing you to experience a deep calm. Because all your energies aren't being drained from you in nervous tension, you will feel more energized as well.

  Rhodiola is available in capsules, tablets, and dried leaf form for a fragrant, comforting, healing tea.

- *Siberian Ginseng*...is one of the most potent whole-body tonics you can use. And when your body is stressed from month to month by PMS you can use a good tonic to build a foundation of well-being. Though it takes two to three weeks for this herb to work, its supportive effects are strong and lasting. There are several kinds of Siberian ginseng, and you should make sure that one of its scientific names—*Eleuthero* or *E. senticosus*—appears on the label, as many substitutes and impostors are being used in its place. The *authentic* Siberian ginseng is known to fortify against long-term stress, and it helps keep blood pressure steady.

  Siberian ginseng comes in capsules and extract, but in root form it makes a great tonic tea.

- *Skullcap*...Does PMS cause you to experience sleep disturbances, nervous hypertension, stress headaches, mood swings? Or all of the above? If so, then skullcap is a good choice.

  This next bit of information may not endear the herb skullcap to you, but in seventeenth-century Europe it was known as "mad dog herb" because it was effective in calming animals with rabies. (Your husband, boyfriend, or boss does not have to know this. Why give them ammunition?)

  Seriously...skullcap is very effective as a headache reliever and as a calming herb when hormonally induced anxiety is rocking your world.

  Skullcap comes in extract or dried in capsule form.

  Note: Skullcap can have strong sedative effects. You should not drive after taking this herb.

- *St. John's wort*...is widely used today to relieve anxiety, treat mood swings, and alleviate mild to moderate depression. Researchers believe that its active compounds—*hypericin, pseudohypericin*, and *hyperforin*—may assist in neurotransmissions within your brain. Thus, the anti-anxiety and anti-depressant effects.

You should note that St. John's wort, like any herbal remedy, takes some time to reach therapeutic levels in your body—up to three weeks. If depression is severe or lasting, or if herbal remedies do not help, you should see a healthcare professional for help. Depression is a serious problem affecting your health and your relationships—your life—and it should never be ignored.

St. John's wort is taken as a tea, in capsules, and in extract.

Note: You should not rely on St. John's wort as your main course of treatment if you are experiencing panic attacks or if you are seriously depressed. It should not be taken if you are using MAO inhibitors, and it does not react well with certain protease inhibitors. Also, this herb is known to cause skin hyper-sensitivity and may increase the danger and damage of sunburn. St. John's wort may also affect the metabolism of Clozaril, Coumadin, Elavil, Haldol, Theo-Dur, Tofranil, Zyflo, and Zyprexa.

- **Valerian**...has become a popular sleep aid because it naturally quiets the mind and induces deep sleep. Its other benefit to women with PMS is that it's a wonderful relaxant, and thus relieves cramps.

Note: Valerian is known to react with barbiturate drugs and should not be taken if you are using drugs in the barbiturate family. If you are taking benzodiazapene drugs like Ativan, Valium, or Xanax you should not use this herb. Valerian should not be used during pregnancy. It also affects the metabolism of Clozaril, Coumadin, Elavil, Haldol, Theo-Dur, Tofranil, Zyfol, and Zyprexa. Finally, you should not drive after taking Valerian.

- **White Willow Bark**...is another powerful, natural inflammatory. Its active ingredient is salycilin so it acts gently to relieve headaches, much the same as meadowsweet.

- *Yarrow*…is another herb with anti-cramping properties. Its therapeutic benefits also include the ability to fight bladder infections and stimulate digestion.

  Yarrow comes in capsules and in extract form.

The Hormone Shelf

Many traditional PMS symptoms—from depression, to moodiness, to severe cramps—are rooted in hormonal fluctuations.

Studies have advanced our knowledge about natural supplements that can help to regulate hormonal production. In fact, there are just a few you should consider. Mostly, they act as "precursors"—that is, building-block substances that help your body produce the hormones or other important biochemicals you need.

- **DHEA (Dehydroepiandrosterone).** This hormone is also used as a natural mood leveler. It can also boost your energy. Because it is a precursor to estrogen (as well as testosterone), it may also help to level out your hormonal cycle as well.

- *Estriol*…is a natural estrogen that does not bind with estrogen receptors at the cellular level. For this reason it will deliver a milder form of estrogen—helpful if you are lacking. But it will not act like a growth hormone, promoting breast tissue growth.

  Many women use estriol suppositories or creams if they are experiencing vaginal dryness or discomfort during intercourse. You should experiment until you find the lowest amount that gives you the results you want.

  This is a substance you may want to remember and return to later because it has even more benefits for postmenopausal women, including helping you keep your bone-density intact.

℞ HOMEOPATHY

～

Homeopathy has been dismissed by many in the American medical community even though it has long been in wide use in much of the rest of the world. Perhaps one reason it's dismissed in "highly scientific" approaches to medicine is that homeopathy links spiritual and emotional conditions to physical symptoms. Obviously, this can be overdone and misused. But as we rediscover those mind-body-spirit connections, people are turning back to homeopathy and finding it effective.

It is featured here only in brief because it's important that you work with a professional trained in homeopathy. Some people claim to find relief by using homeopathic remedies on their own without guidance. But the substances must often be used in combinations, and the doses need to be finely adjusted to offer the maximum benefit.

If you decide to try homeopathic remedies, you may wish to ask about

- **Aconitum**...which helps when stress is causing your period to be late
- **Cimicifuga**...if cramps are intense, almost like labor...and you're anxious or depressed
- **Colocynthis**...if cramps are severe and accompanied by anger
- **Lachesis**...if you suffer from headaches, breast tenderness, ovarian pain, and abandonment anxieties
- **Magnesia phosphorica**...for spasmodic cramps and bloating
- **Pulsatilla**...if you're sad or depressed, and your period is irregular
- **Sepia**...if you have lower back pain, menstrual cramps, or pressure in your reproductive organs

To locate a qualified homeopath in your area, you may wish to contact The American Institute of Homeopathy at (703) 246-9501.

- *Progesterone Cream.* Because excess levels of estrogen are the most prevalent cause of certain PMS symptoms—especially irritability and mood swings—some naturopaths recommend using progesterone cream to keep your hormones in balance.

   The cream can be applied to your breasts or abdomen daily for a month to build to the therapeutic "base" level. Then use it every month after that. Start on day 12 of your cycle, and stop when menstruation begins.

   Some pharmacies may have this cream available, or you may wish to get it through a naturopathic physician.

- *5-HTP* (**5-Hydroxytryptophan**)…is actually a precursor to an amino acid, not a hormone, which your body needs to regulate mood. It's widely used in the self-treatment of depression. This supplement increases your body's production of tryptophan, which in turn boosts your brain's production of that mood-stabilizing neurotransmitter chemical, serotonin.

The Mineral Shelf

There are only a few minerals and trace minerals you need if you're suffering from PMS. But it's *very important* that you get them.

If you're eating a great diet that counters the effects of PMS, such as the one outlined in the previous chapter, you may be getting the minerals and trace minerals you need. Unfortunately, all the stresses of contemporary life work to rapidly deplete our bodies of nutrients—and minerals, like vitamins, are drained rapidly. It most definitely does not hurt—and it's very likely to help—if you supplement with…

- *Calcium, Potassium, and Magnesium.* These three minerals are best taken together, because each affects the body's ability to use the others.

   Calcium and potassium work together to help relax cramps and reduce bloating.

Add magnesium, which maintains healthy levels of neuro-transmitters in the brain responsible for maintaining a level mood, and you guard against anxiety attacks, as well.

- *Chromium.* Chromium is one of those trace minerals we need in only tiny amounts—not even in milligrams, but in *micro*grams. However, even 200 micrograms of chromium a day will help to regulate your blood sugar, reducing irritability.

- *Zinc.* Many of us take zinc at the first signs of cold or flu. This trace mineral is important to many bodily functions, and our bodies sorely miss it when stress or a poor diet leech it from our systems.

For women suffering with PMS-related anxiety, an extra dose of zinc can be an effective treatment.

The Vitamin Shelf

Even if you eat a healthy diet, you can be vitamin-deficient for many different reasons. Stress is one reason your body can quickly deplete itself of vitamins—and PMS is a major stressor. Without the help of vitamins, your glands will not produce hormones properly, your nervous system goes into overload, and in short order, you feel terrible physically, your emotions are crashing, and you can even find it hard to concentrate. You are anxious, tired, and utterly drained.

Here are some of the main vitamins that can help boost you back to balance when PMS is stressing your body to the max.

- *B-Complex* (The "Stress Buffers"). The whole family of B-complex vitamins are among nature's most potent stress-reducers. They boost immunity, keep the nervous system functioning, help translate food energy to our cells, and much more. Unfortunately, they drain from our bodies rapidly when we're under physical or emotional strain.

Because you need them and they're water soluble (meaning your body eliminates any excess of these vitamins through urination), you may want to take more than the recommended

PREVENTING YEAST

∼

When the environment inside a woman's vagina changes, that is, when the pH changes from acidic to basic, the conditions are right for a yeast infection *(candida albicans)* to take over.

Many women are aware that using **acidophilus** can help restore the right interior balance. This promotes the growth of healthy bacteria, which then re-take the territory and replace the yeast bacteria. Acidophilus can be taken in capsule form or can be found in yogurts and milk products that use "active cultures." (Non-dairy versions are also available.)

But did you know there are other natural supplements you can use if acidophilus loses its effectiveness for you? They include...

citrus extract

caprylic acid

tanalbit (tannins, with zinc)

You should also know that certain foods should be on your forbidden list during a yeast infection. These include

alcohol

chocolate

sugar

because they promote the overgrowth of *candida.*

daily allowance on days when your PMS symptoms are the worst and running you down, starting at 100 milligrams a day.

- *Vitamin B₃ (Niacin).* Mainly, niacin improves our cells' ability to receive energy from our foods. Even better for PMS sufferers, it offers significant relief from menstrual cramps.

- *Vitamin B₆ (Pyroxidine)*…also aids in relieving cramps. Beyond that, it relieves tenderness in the breasts and prevents water retention by acting as a natural diuretic. B_6 has wonderful mood-balancing properties, too. It lowers homocysteine levels, which can cause confused thinking when unchecked. And it offers an antidepressant benefit by boosting the level of serotonin in your brain.

  Some experts suggest taking up to 300 milligrams of B_6 as a therapeutic dose.

- *Vitamin B₁₂ (Cobalamin)*. B_{12} helps your liver to deactivate excess estrogen, thus helping to keep your hormone levels stable.

- *Vitamin E.* The most immediate benefit of Vitamin E is that it helps reduce cramping. But if low estrogen production is a problem, Vitamin E can become your friend. Estrogen also plays an important role in keeping your vaginal lining healthy.

  As noted earlier, when the vaginal environment changes its pH balance—from acidic to alkaline—healthy micro-organisms die, and infectious ones such as yeast take over. Vitamin E helps keep your pH balance in the healthy zone.

  Finally, if night sweats are a problem, Vitamin E (often in higher doses) is frequently suggested by naturopaths as a way to control them. You should experiment by starting at 200 IU (International Units) of E a day when you're symptomatic, and slowly build up until you find the dose that works for you.

  Note: Vitamin E acts as a blood thinner, and you should consult with your physician before using it if you are on medications such as Coumadin, Warfarin, or other blood-thinning prescription drugs. Also, you should not use high doses of Vitamin E before or after surgery.

The Scent of Relief

In recent years, "aromatherapy" has evolved from a little known "fad" to mainstream acceptance. Little kiosks in shopping malls sell vials of essential oils. Health food stores feature racks. Each oil is reputed to treat a specific problem—be it a mood disorder or a physical ailment.

Some argue that most of the scents, themselves, have little or no effectiveness. The only benefit, they say, comes from having a pleasant aroma wafting in the air, causing us to inhale more deeply. It's the *deep breathing* that's important, they say, because that in itself cleanses the body of toxins and triggers the deep-relaxation response.

So even if essential oils *only* cause us to breathe deeply, more regularly...wouldn't that be an important reason to use them? Most of us fell out of the habit of breathing properly sometime right after infancy. And learning to breathe deeply again is an advantage for many health problems—including PMS.

Practitioners, including naturopaths and trained herbalists, insist that aromatherapy works because it stimulates the liminal system. They say the scents of certain oils are known to benefit symptoms that accompany PMS—such as mood swings, depression, digestive problems, cramps, sleeplessness, agitation, and more.

Here are some of the most useful fragrances of benefit to PMS sufferers...

- **For mood swings, depression, or anxiety:** bergamot, geranium, rose, and/or ylang-ylang oils

- **For cramps or nausea:** clary sage, lavender, and/or sandalwood oils

- **For hormonal balance:** clary sage oil

- **To promote menstrual flow:** cypress, chamomile, jasmine, lavender, and/or melissa oils

If you become pregnant, you should *not* use the following essential oils: basil, bergamot, cypress, geranium, hyssop, marjoram, melissa, peppermint, sage, thyme, or wintergreen. Check with an aromatherapy expert before using any essential oil during pregnancy.

R✗

CHECK IT OUT

∼

Because some supplements may cause negative reactions in some consumers, it's always best to *read labels carefully*. In addition, Web sites now exist where you can look up information about supplement manufacturers and how their products rate compared to others.

One such site is www.consumerlab.com. The Dietary Supplement Quality Initiative (DSQI) also reviews natural supplements and makes its findings available to the public. Read up on the latest studies on their Web site: www.dsqi.org.

6

Getting Your Body on Your Side

Two older women, both post-menopausal, were talking over lunch. One said wistfully, "I miss being young, don't you?" The friend glanced down at her own chest, now headed toward the sunset position, and laughed wryly. "Are you kidding? Look at me—I'm sagging. Boy, do I miss my old figure and the attention I got. But, honey," she went on, "my periods were a *nightmare*. So, would I go back to *that*? Truthfully, I'd rather *die!*"

Isn't the point of menstruation to create conditions in your body that allow new life to be created? If that's so, then why does it *feel* like your body is bent on destroying you and your little dog, Toto, too?

It doesn't have to be that way.

Your Body Can Become Your Friend Again

You can use your body as an ally in the art of controlling PMS.

Sure, you may want to take a vacation from your body two or three weeks of every month. But because that isn't going to happen you can use some important strategies that will help you keep your physical symptoms in check.

Numerous studies show the strong relationship between health and physical activity. A toned and active body is healthier all-around and far less likely to become sick...and, *if* we get sick, we bounce back more quickly from every sort of ailment or physical distress. If you're active—meaning that you're engaged in a reasonable level of physical activity three or more times a week—you will have:

→ a better metabolism and better digestion

→ better hormone production and regulation

→ more energy instead of fatigue

→ less muscle stiffness, aches, and joint injuries

→ fewer headaches

→ a stronger immune system

→ a more positive mental attitude *and* a lighter spirit

Along with exercise and activity, there are simple techniques you can also use to relieve your body of PMS symptoms.

What follows are some of the most effective strategies you can use.

Best Body Strategies

Strategy #1: Make a Commitment to Your Self

If you're like most women—especially working women and those with families and homes to care for—taking care of your physical body…beyond the basics…comes last on the list. After all that work and all those demands, who has time or energy left to exercise or dance or enjoy outdoor activity?

You *need* to make a commitment to yourself.

Do This:

1. Make your health and well-being a priority.

Life is much better when you live it in a body that functions at its best.

2. Make a written list of your general health goals and affirmations.

So much of what you get in life is determined by what you set your will to accomplish. If you make no commitment to your well-being, then your health will slide gradually downhill. Writing down a goal in the form of an affirmation, like those that follow, will keep you focused:

"I am maintaining a healthy balance in body, mind, and spirit."

"I am practicing good mental and spiritual disciplines. I am eating right every day. I am working out regularly."

Writing goal affirmations in the present tense helps you sense the "do it now/don't put it off" importance of the words. It will also help you return much more quickly to the pathway of the small, daily disciplines that lead you back to your goals on those days when you miss. There is force and energy, a "no matter what" determination in training yourself to say, "I *am* doing this."

Posting these goal affirmations where you can see them daily reminds you to keep your well-being up near the top of your priority list.

As one of your goal affirmations, determine to work out physically. Choose an intensity of physical activity—from light to more aggressive.

- **Design a workout plan that fits your goals and lifestyle…** and schedule it into your week as a top priority. You'll be amazed how other priorities fall in place around it.

- **Redesign your workout plan from time to time** so it doesn't become boring. You may wish to increase its intensity, too.

A workout buddy or two can also help keep you motivated. But don't make your workouts dependent on whether or not the others show up. (You *know* they're always running late!)

Strategy #2: A Good Stretch

You roll out of bed, slide into slippers and robe…and stretch. Feels great, doesn't it? You stimulate deep breathing and release stress, triggering that important deep-relaxation response. Toxins are expressed from your muscles. Joints and tendons are loosened. Blood-flow increases and your metabolism wakes up. *All that* begins with a simple stretch.

Stretching is one of the easiest and most underrated physical regimens you can use to improve physical and mental health.

You can experience wonderful health benefits just by starting or ending your day with the following simple stretching regimen. Most of these moves can also be done at the office, too, and a few can even be used to de-stress and refresh you while stuck in a car in traffic or when you feel a tension headache or sick stomach coming on.

Do This:

1. Sit in an open space on the floor...or in a chair if you need back support.

If you're sitting on the floor, move your legs until they're comfortably apart.

℞

A TOUCH OF LIGHT

~

Our whole being craves sunlight. If we don't get enough of it, unhappy things happen.

Our brains produce too little of key hormones, and our mood slips. Our bodies fail to produce vitamin D and cannot use the vitamin K we get from foods, and as a result, our immune function drops.

No wonder so many women suffer from depression, colds, flus...and no wonder PMS symptoms are worse in the colder, darker months.

One good solution is to purchase full-spectrum lighting, available in health food stores, some discount stores, and pet stores.

An even better solution is to get yourself outside for a brisk walk every day during daylight hours. Even a ten-minute walk in winter's weaker sunlight restores your body to normal functioning.

Besides giving your heart and lungs a small workout, you'll get the touch of light you need to help restore well-being.

Begin by loosening your hips, the back of your thighs, and buttocks. These are the largest muscle groups in your body. When you were a baby in utero—think about how you were packaged then—these were firm and flexible. The more you've aged, the less you've stretched and firmed these important muscles. (Is it any wonder they're stiff and a bit "softer" now?)

- Slowly lower your torso toward one knee...then the other. Feel the muscles in your hips, buttocks, and the back of you thighs stretch.

- After you stretch each side out, take a cleansing breath. In slowly through your nose...out in a puff through your mouth. (Continue this after each set of recommended stretches.)

As with every move suggested here, go *slowly* and *gently*. Never force a stretch, or you may harm muscles and hamstrings. Use your fingers to knead tight muscles as you go along.

The muscles in this area of your body have been called "the second heart," because when they stretch and pump they increase overall circulation dramatically. And if you want to work against the aging, stiffening, and sagging process, these are important muscle groups to keep limber and toned.

2. Loosen up your neck.

Never roll your head in a circle to stretch the neck muscles as it's very easy to damage the delicate vertebrae, disks, and nerves in your neck. Instead,

- Tip your head to the left as if to touch your ear to your shoulder. Feel the tendons and muscles on your right side stretch. Repeat on the right side.

- From the head-up starting position, tip your head forward and touch your chin to your chest. Feel the back of your neck relax.

Keeping your neck loose and free of muscle knots will prevent these muscles from pinching on the nerves passing through them, which sends "tension" and "pain" signals up through your face and head...resulting in that tired-around-the eyes or dull-headachy feeling.

3. Loosen your shoulders.

This continues the process of releasing tight trigger points, expressing lactic acid, and increasing blood flow in the neck, shoulders, and torso.

- Raise your left shoulder to your ear, then roll it forward and down. (You may hear "clunks" in your shoulder blade. If they're painless, don't worry.) The goal is to feel the muscles between your shoulder blade and spine stretch and relax. Repeat, using your right shoulder.

4. Loosen your chest and abdomen.

- Extend your arms with your elbows locked and palms down, and place one hand on the back of the other.

- Slowly raise your arms till they're pointing straight up. As you do, breathe in and feel your diaphragm fill. Reach for the sky and feel your chest and abdominal muscles stretch.

- Move your arms a little farther back, till they're behind your head. Clasp hands. Using your right hand, draw your left arm down to the right and feel the muscles along your left side stretch. Repeat, using your left hand...and make your right side happy.

  You are *remembering to breathe through the stretches, aren't you?*

5. Loosen your calves and quadriceps.

- Straighten your left leg and point your toes. Feel your shins stretch. Repeat on the right. Push your left heel out, feeling your calf stretch. Now, the right.

- Grab your left ankle. Slowly draw your leg back behind you and feel the quads on the front of your legs stretch. (Don't overextend your knee joint.) Relax. Repeat for the benefit of your right leg.

You've just completed a full-body stretch that's released stress from your muscles and stimulated your metabolism and blood flow. It's also released healthy endorphins into your body that are helping regulate hormone production. And it's taken you one step down the path to that goal of a healthier, more youthful *you.*

THE 8000-YEAR-OLD WONDER

∼

For some 8000 years a whole range of exercises based on stretching and then holding postures has been used to promote total health in many parts of the world. Yoga builds youthful strength and endurance, improves mental ability, encourages spiritual growth...and it offers more specialized benefits for women with PMS. For instance, it helps release endorphins, those calming, health-regulating hormones, and it relieves tensions throughout the body—especially in those deep abdominal muscles involved in cramping.

If you want to go beyond the simple stretching routine previously recommended, you can easily find instructional yoga classes, books, and videos. Many come *sans* eastern philosophies, leaving you to enjoy just the amazing health benefits.

Strategy #3: Get to the Point...with Acupressure

Let's say your PMS symptoms have hit overnight. Your muscles are stiff and achy. You feel dull or even excruciating pain in your back, shoulders, neck, or head. Maybe you know that the more the day goes on, the more likely it is that this tense, achiness is going to zero-in on your stomach...and cramps are just a few hours away.

Acupressure is a great way to relieve headaches and muscle cramping. Because it triggers the deep-relaxation response, it also has the marvelous side benefit of restoring a focus of inner calm accompanied by an overall sense of well-being.

To use acupressure, simply use your finger tips or knuckles to explore the nerve pathways in various parts of your body...where you'll find that muscles have tensed at certain points, clenching the nerves that pass through them. These are called trigger points because they will trigger the next muscle to clench...and the next, and the next. It's this clenching that pinches your nerves, decreases blood flow, and leaves you with pain radiating all around that area of your body.

Following are charts that will help you quickly locate trigger points that are important for relieving pain and distress in various parts of your body—in your head, neck, shoulders, back, and abdomen. You can reach most of them yourself...but of course it's nicer if someone else works on them for you.

Relieving Headaches and Neck Aches

Figure 1 shows two sets of trigger points—responsible for headaches—which are located on the fine bones of your face. These are located around your eyes (1) and along both your cheek and jaw bones (2). **Figure 2** shows you a side view of Figure 1...plus more sets, located at the base of your skull and running down the back of your neck right beside the spinal vertebrae (3) and down the sides of your neck to the tops of your shoulders (4).

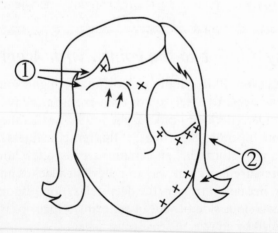

Figure 1

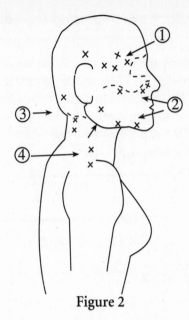

Figure 2

Relieving Headaches and Upper Back Pains

A set of trigger points around the surface of your shoulder blades, shown in **Figure 3**, also generates head and neck aches (**5**). And a set down along your backbone to its midpoint creates middle and upper back pain (**6**).

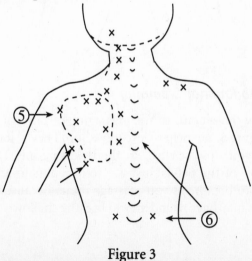

Figure 3

Relieving Lower Back and Radiating Leg Pains

Look at **Figure 4** and you'll see that yet another set of trigger points is located along the top of the underside of the pelvic ridge, just above the buttocks (7). These mostly generate lower back pain, but you may also be surprised to find a headache radiating from this far south, up along your spine to the back of your neck and even around to your temples! You may also find shooting leg pains radiating from these trigger points.

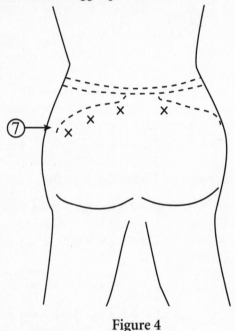

Figure 4

Relieving Abdominal Cramping

And now those cramps. Yes, massaging certain trigger points, shown in **Figure 5**, can help relieve those, too. They're located at the outsides of your lowest ribs...in the ticklish zone. They're also along the top of the pelvis, just where it begins to angle down. (Remember to breathe as you massage these. Because this area is sensitive you may have a tendency to breathe shallowly.)

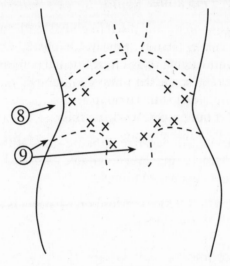

Figure 5

Strategy #4: Walk Out of the PMS zone

When you need to shake the stresses and moods of PMS, knowing how to walk yourself out of the "PMS zone" will help you (and anyone who happens to be in your zone, too). Walking is a low-impact way to make your muscles work out toxins, stimulate your metabolism, trigger normal hormonal production, and oxygenate the blood. (It's also a great mini-vacation from house or office work. What's not to like?)

Do This:

1. Establish two or three walking routes.

Make sure you have an easy route for those tougher days when it's not wise to push yourself physically, another for days when you're feeling so-so, and a third for the days you're feeling good and just need to keep your walking regimen going. Choose routes that will give you changes in scenery if you can.

2. Establish a "PMS zone."

This is where good mental disciplines that teach you to refocus your mind come in very handy. (Review Chapter 2.) On days when your symptoms are driving you nuts, set mental boundaries around it. Your zone may be "inside the walls of this house," or "at the edge of the property," or "inside this work place."

When you set out on your walk, do this:

- Tell yourself, "All negative thinking stops at the boundary I've set—including every agitated, worried, depressed, stressed, or aggravated thought."

- Tell yourself, "I'll focus instead on whatever is good, lovely, nice, high, or inspiring."

3. Walk your course.

Any time a thought returns that would produce a negative mindset or darken your spirit, gently turn back to positive thoughts. You can also take your mind out-of-gear by refocusing on your breathing.

4. As you return, shrink your PMS zone.

Women sometimes put too much pressure on themselves to be "nice" all the time. Don't pressure yourself to be a plaster saint with a painted-on smile if you're feeling crampy, bloated, and headachy. On the other hand, you also don't need to slaughter anyone who accidentally steps on your tail.

As you return to your house or workplace, try these PMS containment ideas:

- Take three minutes to write down what's gotten to you so far today…or this week. Write one positive, reasonable thing you can do to resolve the tension or annoyance you feel.

- Compose a simple statement or two that becomes your script when people pressure or bug you: "I'm really feeling awful today, and so I'm not handling pressure well. I'm

doing the best I can right now, so just go lightly with me."
Or even, "Something's bothering me today. [You don't have
to say what.] If I'm snappish or abrupt, don't take it per-
sonally."

Learning how to walk out of your personal PMS zone will
help you feel better *and* regain control of life on those
rough days.

HERBAL BATHS
∼

Exercise, eh? Physical activity, eh? Maybe some days you
can…and maybe on other days you just *can't.*

Whether it comes after a good workout or a rough day, an
herbal bath soothes physical symptoms such as muscle
cramps, digestive discomforts, and headaches. It also calms
you and lifts your mood. It's also a wonderfully simple and
inexpensive way to pamper yourself.

Draw a tub of warm, not hot, water, and depending on the
symptoms you need to ease, try one of these two herbal baths.

To ease menstrual discomforts:

2 tablespoons dried chamomile
2 tablespoons dried hops
2 tablespoons dried lavender
2 tablespoons dried rose
(Nix the rose and add 2 tablespoons of eucalyptus if you
feel headachy.)

To stabilize moodswings and lift your spirit:

4 tablespoons dried peppermint
(*or* 2 drops wintergreen essential oil)
4 tablespoons eucalyptus
4 tablespoons dried orange or lemon zest

Unless you really like wiping out the tub and picking wet
leaves off your body, cut the foot off an old pair of pantyhose
or use an old sock as your infusion bag. Add a little soft music,
and you're on your way.

Strategy #5: Workout "Lite"

So you want to up it a notch from stretching? Included in this strategy are activities like *short-course jogging, rollerblading, easy cycling,* and *dancercise.*

A light aerobic workout may be the most strenuous workout you can handle if PMS symptoms are distressing. Believe it or not, even if you are experiencing the worst part of your cycle…and even if you feel fatigued…a light workout can help.

Light aerobic exercise is incredibly rejuvenating. It increases your blood flow and metabolism, which regulates hormonal production and at the same time cleanses your body of both normal toxins and excess hormones. Because it triggers the release of endorphins, it's also a wonderful, natural mood elevator. Additionally, it restores the focus that emotional depression or agitation has scattered.

You will feel the benefits of light aerobic exercise almost immediately—and if you design it into your life regularly, in just two or three weeks (really!) you'll experience a wonderful restoration of youthful energy and vitality. (Who knows, you may be able to kick caffeine after all!)

Strategy #6: Non-Impact Aerobics (NIA)

Many women have discovered the health-restoring benefits of non-impact aerobics. These exercises can be just the ticket if you're prone to serious headaches and can't take the jarring of more strenuous workout routines.

NIA combines stretching with a choreography of fluid motions and proper breathing. The routines can best be described as a blend of aerobics, ballet, muscle toning, *tai chi,* and yoga. This regimen was developed by two aerobics instructors, Debbie and Carlos Rosas, who realized that high-impact aerobics can lead to serious injuries for some and also provides too much of a challenge for people dealing with delicate health conditions. This makes NIA a good choice for women with PMS.

As for physical benefits—NIA increases your metabolism, respiration, heart rate, and also the production of those all-important neurotransmitter chemicals that boost your mood. It also stimulates the adrenal gland, which regulates hormone production, too.

NIA instructors encourage "mental conditioning," too. Some use guided meditations as a way to focus and cleanse the mind of counterproductive thinking. You can also plan your own "mental workout" during NIA exercises, focusing on personal affirmations. Or give your spirit a boost by meditating on favorite scriptures or inspirational thoughts.

Rx

A LITTLE MUSIC
(AND THE RIGHT SHOES, OF COURSE!)
∼

Music has a powerfully therapeutic effect on the whole body. From time immemorial its soothing rhythms and melodies have lulled cranky babies to sleep and stirred souls to love and devotion.

Matching music to whatever light aerobics regimen you choose is one of the secrets to a more effective workout. Music that's slow and fluid works great for stretching. Livelier dance music can give you an added charge of energy while running or cycling. (Just remember to stay alert for traffic!)

Shoes. When you're dancing, jumping, or running your feet are absorbing as much as two or three times your body weight. *So don't buy cheap shoes.* You don't need $150 athletic shoes—but you do need enough cushion and support to help your feet have a nice time while you restore well-being to the rest of your body.

Do This:

1. Check local community centers, gyms, and health clubs to sign up for NIA classes.

When you find a program, schedule it into your week as a top priority.

2. Purchase a recorded version of sacred and inspirational writings or a recording of positive affirmations.

3. As you engage in the NIA routines, let your mind be renewed and your spirit made lighter.

Reaffirm your commitment to your personal well-being.

Strategy #7: Weight Training

Weight training offers many benefits, far beyond the obvious—a well-toned body. Many women enjoy the gentle rigors of light-course weight training these days.

Women with PMS find that keeping up a regimen during their "good weeks" helps relieve physical distresses during the tough days. First, they increase their metabolism, which keeps circulation and respiration at a good pace. Second, the adrenal gland is stimulated, which helps regulate hormone production.

If you're already involved, you need no instructions…and if you aren't, you're better off joining a health club and getting specific instructions on the machines from a trainer. (Yes, you should ask about the trainer's experience.)

As an aid to easing PMS symptoms…

Do This:

1. Develop a good overall workout—one that tones and strengthens your whole body.

Work your upper and lower body on alternate days. If you can work out only one or two days a week, give yourself a little more time and work out your whole body.

Good overall muscle tone helps prevent those nasty little knots from forming at the trigger points, causing stiffness and ugly headaches.

❤ **TARGET HEART-RATES** ❤

Whether you're walking, dancing, or using NIA to boost your body, you'll have the most effective workout if you reach your "target heart rate" and maintain it for at least 30 minutes.

The target heart rate that's right for you is largely dependent on your age. (Remember, though, you always want to consult with your doctor before starting a physical regimen, especially if you have health problems.) The target heart rate represents a range consisting of the minimum and maximum number of heartbeats per minute you want to maintain while working out. You want to reach at least the minimum and not go over the maximum.

If you hit your target heart rate at least three times a week and maintain it for 30 minutes, you have contributed amazingly to your overall health. And women with PMS report a vast decrease in symptoms after establishing a workout routine that helps them hit this target.

Find your target heart-rate here:

Age	Range
Up to 25	117 to 156 beats per minute (20 to 26 beats per 10 seconds)
26 to 35	111 to 148 beats per minute (19 to 25 beats per 10 seconds)
36 to 45	105 to 140 beats per minute (18 to 23 beats per 10 seconds)
46 to 55	99 to 132 beats per minute (17 to 22 beats per 10 seconds)
55 +	93 to 124 beats per minute (16 to 21 beats per 10 seconds)

To check your pulse…Place the index and middle finger of your right hand on your left medial artery, which is that blue "pencil" line running through your wrist at the base of your left thumb.

2. Focus on toning and strengthening your mid-section.

Using the incline benches, either for sit-ups or for inclined presses will help to firm up your stomach muscles. If your stomach is toned, you're less likely to experience cramping from PMS—or you'll recover faster from it if you do.

3. Chart your progress.

Because a woman's life has a cyclical rhythm to it, it can have a subliminal effect on you. You can feel like saying, "I'm stuck in exactly the same place I was last month...and the month before that...and...." Anything you can do to mark progress in any area will help to keep you from slipping into the *I'm-going-nowhere blues.*

Keep a small notebook handy and record the weights you use for each exercise and the number of repetitions you can do. Watching your gains will give your mind and spirit an added boost on those days when your body is tempting you to feel crummy about yourself.

WHY YOU NEED TO REWARD YOURSELF

∼

A reward is just a tangible way to mark an achievement. Sure, it would be nice if other people rewarded us for tasks well-done and progress made...but it would also be nice if they just picked up after themselves all the time. (And when is *that* going to happen?)

A reward is only meaningful if it's attached to a real accomplishment. (Sorry, rewarding yourself with a huge dessert just because it's Friday evening doesn't count.) But when you have made gains in life, you need to see that you're rewarded, even if you reward yourself...for these important reasons:

1. **Most of us are starving for rewards that mark our achievements, whether in words or in the form of an actual prize.** What words do you want to hear? What little, tangible reward would nicely pick up your spirit and be a reminder of what you've accomplished?

2. **A reward gives us good motivation to continue**—especially when you're trying to form a new habit or when the going gets tough.

3. **Rewarding is a habit we can also use to benefit other people** who are just as starved as we are for a kind word of affirmation or a small prize to keep them going.

Know someone who's stingy with praise? Tight-fisted with rewards? You don't want to be like them, do you?

Learn how to have a generous, rewarding spirit—one that can lift others' spirits along with your own.

7

Finding Balance

Throughout this book, we've been emphasizing the need to find balance in your search for freedom from PMS. You're most likely to experience health and overall well-being if you learn how to be healthy in every aspect of your whole person—body, mind, and spirit.

Finding balance—that is, the strategies you need to achieve your healthiest state—is not difficult. But it *does* take a bit of work, and that's where you may need a little help. The usual pattern goes like this:

You buy a book like this one. You read it and pick up one or two items of interest. You try them—for a little while at least. One or two strategies seem to work.

Then you slip a little. You forget that a certain food sends your nerves through the roof. You run out of that herb that really helped. And it's very easy to slip out of the mental and spiritual practices that relieved your deep-level stresses.

There You Are Again

And there you are again, right back in the distress of PMS. If you're tempted to feel badly about yourself—forget it. *Welcome to human nature.*

We all need "prompts"—practical tools that can help us stay on-track with new and healthy changes we want to make in our lives. We need these prompts even if we find changes that really work for our benefit, because our human tendency is always to return to old patterns. We're just that way.

What follows is a simple tool you can use to create healthy new habits, using strategies that work to relieve your PMS symptoms. This tool will help you...

- track PMS symptoms from week to week throughout your cycle

- record strategies you're trying and the benefits they offer you

Physical symptoms, mental stress, and spiritual stress are listed separately for a reason. Often, you may be so focused on one type of symptom—your blistering PMS headaches, for example—that you tend to ignore the fact that you're mentally stressed or down in spirit. "Checking in" with the aspects of your total being will help you get a better picture of the kind of help and support you actually need.

Feel free to make copies of the following pages. Use them to track your symptoms from month to month—also to record which strategies you're using and which ones work for you.

Week One: Menstruation

Your flow begins, and around the fifth day it ends. Hormonal signals from your pituitary gland reach your ovaries and trigger an egg to start maturing. Your uterine lining thickens, preparing to receive the egg, if it's fertilized.

• Physical Symptoms (besides the obvious)_____

_____

• Relief Strategies and Benefits _____

_____

• Dietary Changes and Benefits _____

_____

• Supplements and Benefits _____

_____

• Mental Stresses Encountered _____

_____

• Relief Strategies and Benefits _____

_____

• Spiritual Stresses Recognized _____

_____

• Relief Strategies and Benefits _____

_____

Week Two: Ovulation

Throughout this week, several egg follicles are developing, and one is taking the lead. Estrogen and progesterone production are in high gear, and estrogen in particular reaches its maximum levels in your body. Around day 14, the mature egg begins making its way to your uterus. Often, this is a trouble-free, energized week—but *not* a signal to stop using important health strategies.

- Physical Symptoms _____

  _____

- Relief Strategies and Benefits _____

  _____

- Dietary Changes and Benefits _____

  _____

- Supplements and Benefits _____

  _____

- Mental Stresses Encountered _____

  _____

- Relief Strategies and Benefits _____

  _____

- Spiritual Stresses Recognized _____

  _____

- Relief Strategies and Benefits _____

  _____

Week Three: Preparing for Fertility

Your egg is making its way down the fallopian tube. Progesterone levels rise, causing blood vessels to swell. Your uterine lining is thickening rapidly. Bloating, moodiness, and breast tenderness can set in.

- Physical Symptoms _____

  _____

- Relief Strategies and Benefits _____

  _____

- Dietary Changes and Benefits _____

  _____

- Supplements and Benefits _____

  _____

- Mental Stresses Encountered _____

  _____

- Relief Strategies and Benefits _____

  _____

- Spiritual Stresses Recognized _____

  _____

- Relief Strategies and Benefits _____

  _____

Week Four: End of Your Cycle

If your egg has not been fertilized, it disintegrates. At the end of this week, it will be eliminated with your menstrual flow. PMS symptoms—such as cramps, bloating, moodiness, breast tenderness, and headaches—can remain in full swing.

• Physical Symptoms _____

_____

• Relief Strategies and Benefits _____

_____

• Dietary Changes and Benefits _____

_____

• Supplements and Benefits _____

_____

• Mental Stresses Encountered _____

_____

• Relief Strategies and Benefits _____

_____

• Spiritual Stresses Recognized _____

_____

• Relief Strategies and Benefits _____

_____

Once you've begun to see what works, you can use the information to strike the balance of strategies that help you control PMS. You can also track changes in the pattern of your monthly cycle, noting when symptoms change—and also noting when one strategy loses its effectiveness and you need to replace it with another.

A Final Word...About Caring for You

I have a final, great hope for all women who read this book.

Many of you are doing way too much—placing really high demands on yourselves physically, emotionally, mentally, and spiritually.

Some of you are frustrated and stressed out high achievers who have a hard time cutting yourself any slack. Yours is the car with the bumper sticker that says, "No Whining." If you were in a fairy tale you'd be "the miller's daughter," because no matter how much pressure life dumps on you, you keep thinking you should just be able to spin more gold out of straw.

Others of you feel defeated before you start. You have a million eyes in your head, and they're hypertrained on all those overachievers you just read about. Why oh *why* can't you just be more like them?

Many women I know—the ones who can't stop striving, and the ones who can't stop comparing themselves to the strivers—seem to share some common traits.

Maybe you look back at your grandmother's or great-grandmother's generation, and you see how rough most of those women had it—getting by without modern conveniences, sometimes with far less money, and often with more kids to care for. The bottom line is, you often look at yourself and your struggles and you think, "Who am I to pay so much attention to my personal needs?"

And so you minimize or ignore your needs.

Or you look around you...at your parents, your husband, your kids...and you see all their needs. You focus on what you can do to help them, thinking, "A good [daughter, wife, mother] always takes care of the needs of others." As for focusing on your most important needs...

…once again, you don't.

Let's set the record straight.

Noticing personal need is *not* being whiny, and ignoring personal need is *not* heroic.

Focusing on your need for good self-care is *not* a luxury, and it's *not* the same as being selfish or self-centered. Good self-care raises your total quality of life. The better you care for your needs, the more you make it possible to achieve important personal goals…and the better you are able to care for the people you love.

Making self-care a priority is—for sure—a benefit of living in the times we live in, when more options are available to us. Rest assured, if earlier generations of women had these same options, they would have used them to good benefit.

If you need more than the weekly tracking pages at the front of this chapter…if you need a primary commitment to good self-care to support the important work you're doing…I offer in closing the following personal affirmation. Use it as a starter to create one of your own. Use it as a prayer…. But *do* use it.

Affirmation

I will no longer ignore or minimize my real need for good self-care.

- ~ I will not overlook physical, mental, or spiritual symptoms that cause me distress, imagining they will just go away or telling myself, "Just live with it."

- ~ I will not put off my own needs indefinitely, ignoring myself while serving the needs of others.

- ~ I will not tell myself I cannot afford the money, time, or energy it takes to care for my personal health needs.

Instead, I will make every reasonable effort to become aware of my needs in body, mind, and spirit.

- ~ I will pay attention to my body and listen to its warnings and signals of pain and distress. I will feed it, care for it, and not abuse it by poor eating, alcohol or drugs, or by denying it healthy activity.

~ I will pay attention to my mind and not talk myself out of intuitions about myself and my needs. I will seek help, without shame, when I feel confused, distressed, or obsessive.

~ I will learn to listen to my spirit and understand its cries when I am frustrated, sad, depressed, doubting, or despairing. I will create supportive relationships with people of faith who can help me care for my spirit by keeping confidences and by offering encouragement and redirection without judgment.

I will respect my life because it is the only life I have... and it is God's great gift to me.

Notes

1. See 2 Timothy 1:7.
2. See the New International Version's translation of the verse.
3. Proverbs 15:30, paraphrased.
4. See Proverbs 20:27 KJV.
5. See Psalm 139:13.
6. See Proverbs 3:8.
7. See Matthew 7:1.
8. See Matthew 5:45.

The New Nature Institute

The New Nature Institute was founded in 1999 for the purpose of exploring the connection between personal health and wellness and spirituality, with the Hebrew-Christian tradition as its spiritual foundation.

Drawing upon this tradition, the Institute supports the belief that humankind is created in the image of God. We are each body, mind, and spirit and so intricately connected that each aspect of our being affects the other. If one aspect suffers, our whole being suffers; if all aspects are being supported, we will enjoy a greater sense of well-being.

For this reason, the Institute engages in ongoing research in order to provide up-to-date information that supports a "whole-person" approach to wellness. Most especially, research is focused on the natural approaches to wellness that support health and vitality in the body, the mind, and the spirit.

Healthy Body, Healthy Soul is a series of books intended to complement treatment plans provided by healthcare professionals. They are not meant to be used in place of professional consultations and/or treatment plans.

Along with creating written materials, the New Nature Institute also presents seminars, workshops, and retreats on a range of topics relating to spirituality and wellness. These can be tailored for corporate, spiritual community, or general community settings.

For information contact:

The New Nature Institute
Attn: David Hazard
P.O. Box 568
Round Hill, Virginia 20142
(540) 338-7032
Exangelos@aol.com

Books by David Hazard
in the Healthy Body, Healthy Soul Series

Reducing Stress
Breaking Free from Depression
Building Cancer Resistance
Relieving Headaches and Migraines
Controlling PMS
Managing Your Allergies